COMMUNITY ART: CREATIVE APPROACHES TO PRACTICE

JILL M. CHONODY, EDITOR

COMMUNITY ART: CREATIVE APPROACHES TO PRACTICE

JILL M. CHONODY, EDITOR

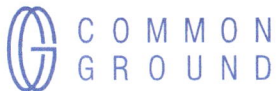

COMMON GROUND

First published in 2014 in Champaign, Illinois, USA
by Common Ground Publishing LLC
as part of the Art in Society book series

Library of Congress Cataloging-in-Publication Data

Community art : creative approaches to practice / Jill M. Chonody, editor.
    pages cm
Includes bibliographical references and index.
ISBN 978-1-61229-565-7 (pbk : alk. paper) -- ISBN 978-1-61229-566-4 (pdf)
1. Arts--Therapeutic use. 2. Creation (Literary, artistic, etc.)--Therapeutic use. 3. Creative ability.
4. Community mental health services. I. Chonody, Jill M., editor.

RC489.A72C66 2014
615.8'5156--dc23

2014029479

Table of Contents

Acknowledgements

I am grateful to my partner Tavis for all of his ongoing love and support. I am also grateful to my colleagues, friends, and family who have contributed to this book in many different ways, including writing, feedback, and cheerleading.

Contributor Biographies

Jill M. Chonody, MSW, PhD, LCSW is an associate professor of social work at Indiana University Northwest where she teaches social work practice and research methodology courses. She is also an adjunct research fellow at the University of South Australia where she has ongoing research collaborations in psychology. She researches issues related to attitudes, in particular ageism, and is interested in scale development and psychometrics. She also seeks to incorporate photography as a research methodology as well as a creative approach to practice. Jill previously worked as a therapist for eight years in both outpatient and inpatient psychiatric facilities.

Jill Amitrani Welsh, MSW earned her Master's of Social Work at Temple University. She is an adjunct faculty member in the Sociology department and the assistant director of the Faith-Justice Institute at Saint Joseph's University.

Barbra Teater, PhD, MSW is an associate professor of social work at the College of Staten Island, The City University of New York. She has over six years of experience in practicing social work as a child and family therapist, medical social worker, and in tobacco cessation and prevention. Barbra teaches community practice, social work theories and methods, and communication and interviewing skills. Barbra's research interests include health and wellbeing among older adults, the social and economic impacts of community-based programs, and creative approaches to social work practice. Barbra works closely with the *Golden Oldies Charity*, which is a singing group for older adults in the southwest of England.

Lisa Hodge is a counsellor at Uniting Communities and a sessional staff member in the School of Psychology, Social Work, and Social Policy at the University of South Australia. Having recently submitted her doctoral thesis, Lisa's primary research interests include eating disorders and mental health more broadly as well as child sexual abuse.

Fiona Buchanan, PhD is a lecturer in social work with the School of Psychology, Social Work and Social Policy at the University of South Australia. She has many years of experience as a critical social worker in women's services and community health services in the UK and Australia. Fiona's research interests include violence against women, child welfare, relationships between women and children, maternal protectiveness, knowledge based in emotions, and using arts in research.

Donna Wang, PhD is an assistant professor in the Social Work department at Long Island University in Brooklyn. Her scholarly interests are gerontological social work education, alternative treatments for mental well-being in older adults, and mental health treatment of ethnic minorities. Her teaching interests include gerontology, research, and human behavior. She has over ten years of practice experience in the areas of child welfare, older adults services, and non-profit management and program development.

Emily Nussdorfer, MA, BC-DMT earned her Master's in dance movement therapy from MCP Hahnemann University in 2001, is a board-certified Dance Movement Therapist (DMT), and has been providing DMT services to diverse populations of all ages for 13 years. A former actress with the Living Theatre in NYC and Pennsylvania State Council of the Arts teaching artist, she has conducted workshops and residencies in dance and creative theater to children and adults for over 20 years. In 2003, she launched the *Girls on the Move* program and founded Moving Creations, Inc. (www.movingcreations inc.org) to support the empowerment needs of adolescent girls living in high-risk inner city Philadelphia communities. She is currently teaching a series of workshops in dance and social change at Bryn Mawr College and has taught workshops in the healing power of dance at Drexel University, Gwynedd Mercy College, West Chester University, University of Pennsylvania, and University of the Arts.

Tina Maschi, PhD is an associate professor at the Fordham University Graduate School of Social Service in New York City, President of the National Organization of Forensic Social Work, and Executive Director of the *Be the Evidence Project*. Tina is also a licensed clinical social worker with over 15 years of experience in correctional health, mental health, and social care in prison and community settings. Her research and practice interests are at the intersection of aging, trauma, mental health, and social justice as well as social work and interprofessional education and workforce development. She is a professional musician and artist and incorporates the use of the arts in research, practice, and advocacy efforts.

Thalia MacMillan, PhD is an assistant professor and mentor of community and human services in the Center for Distance Learning at SUNY Empire State College. She received her PhD. in social work from Fordham University. Thalia has taught courses on disabilities, social research methods, program evaluation, social policy analysis and implementation, assessment and diagnosis, chemical addiction, stress coping, and statistical methods. She currently teaches in several learning modalities, including online, blended learning, and face-to-face. Her professional and academic interests are in online learning, mentoring adult learners, mental health, disabilities, and gerontology.

Keith A. Anderson, MSW, PhD is an associate professor and Hartford Faculty Scholar in the College of Social Work at The Ohio State University. Prior to his current position, Keith was a clinical social worker at The Washington Home, a nursing home and hospice in Washington, DC. His scholarship focuses on the health and well-being of older adults and their caregivers, understanding and improving quality of life in long-term care, informal helping networks, and end-of-life issues. He currently serves as the editor of the *End of Life Care Series* published by Columbia University Press. Keith is also an active outdoorsman and wooden boat devotee.

Jennie R. Babcock, MSW, LISW-S is the undergraduate studies director at The Ohio State University College of Social Work. She came to the College in 2004 as a field coordinator and has teaching experience in generalist practice and ethics. Prior to her position at the College of Social Work, Jennie was a clinical social worker at The Ohio State University Wexner Medical Center, where she worked with children, adolescents, and their families on the inpatient psychiatric unit. Jennie is also an avid gardener and animal enthusiast.

Priscilla Dunk-West, PhD is senior lecturer in social work at Flinders University. She has practiced as a social worker and later as an academic in both England and Australia. In 2011, she co-edited *Sexuality and Sexual Identities in Social Work: Research and Reflections from Women in the Field* (Ashgate) and is the co-author of *Sociological Social Work* (2013, Ashgate). In her latest book, *How to be a Social Worker: A Critical Guide for Students* (2013, Palgrave Macmillan), she applies George Herbert Mead's theory of self to social work identity. She continues to teach social work students and researches in the areas of professional self-making, sexuality, and gender and intimacy.

Caron J. Leader, MSW, LCSW, ACSW, partner and psychotherapist, graduated from the University of Cincinnati with a Bachelor of Arts degree and received her Master of Social Work degree from the University of Southern Indiana. Caron worked at the AIDS Resource Group of Evansville, Southwestern Behavioral Healthcare, and Catholic Charities before starting in private practice. She is also an adjunct professor at the University of Southern Indiana. Caron treats children, adolescents, and adults and has extensive training in Expressive Play Therapy, Cognitive Behavioral Therapy, and Client-Directed Outcome-Informed therapy. Caron utilizes this training to help people with anxiety, AD/HD, depression, grief, and other common life problems.

Wilson Main is a lecturer in Film/TV at the University of South Australia, a producer/writer/director of over 800 broadcast episodes of television, and a consultant to numerous film and television projects around the world. His production work has involved USA, UK, New Zealand, Asia, Africa, and Europe. The work has included children's television, social and wildlife documentary, and factual television. His programs have been broadcast on the Nine and Ten Networks in Australia, PBS (USA), Leoning TV (China), NHK (Japan) and many other international outlets. He has consulted at various times to BBC Worldwide, CCTV (China), Londolozi (South Africa) Kojo Productions (Australia), Fruit Ninja (Australia), Papageno Productions (NZ) and numerous others. He is currently completing a PhD on the barriers to producing television programs featuring female protagonists.

Carolyn Bilsborow, PhD completed her Doctor of Philosophy in the School of Communication, International Studies, and Languages at the University of South Australia in 2013. She teaches in the course *Introduction to Digital Media, Drama Production,* and *Documentary Production*. She has also worked as a Research Assistant, supporting Federal Government-funded projects through researching and producing short video productions. In 2009, Carolyn produced two documentaries for the *2008 Northern Summit,* which won the *University of South Australia's Chancellor's Award for Community Engagement.* Carolyn's research interests are in digital media, particularly documentary production and practice-based research.

Russell Fewster, PhD has directed theatre for 30 years including work with professional actors, acting students, and young people. He studied at Ecole Jacques Lecoq in Paris, and he completed a Masters by Research in rehearsal decision making at the Centre for Performance Studies at the University of Sydney. In 2010, he completed his practice led research PhD at the University of Melbourne, examining the use of projection in performance. He is the program director for the Media Arts Program and lectures in drama and film at the University of South Australia. In 2012, he directed *Perish the Thought* a moving stage portrayal of the effects of dementia on family life. He is currently developing several creative works including film and theatre projects.

Susan Harris is an arts practitioner, educator, author, and playwright, whose work includes social justice related projects. She holds a Graduate Diploma in Community Cultural Development: Arts Based Practice, and a Master of Arts Degree in Communications Management. Susan facilitates community, children's, and youth workshops and has undertaken 75 arts based residencies since 1984. She is a private service provider for Professional Development for the Department of Education and Child Development in Australia and has lectured in World Puppetry for the University of South Australia for 18 years. Susan has produced a series of CDs and books as an Early Childhood education resource; and has authored *A Special Place: Caring for a Parent with Alzheimer's – The Journey,* which she adapted for theatre performance as the play *Perish the Thought.* Both were produced as a voice for carers. Susan also facilitates workshops for parents on *Children and Literacy through the Arts.*

Laura Wernick, PhD, LMSW, MPA is an assistant professor at Fordham University School of Social Service. She completed her PhD in social work and political science, and a graduate certificate in women's studies at the University of Michigan. Her research examines how people can work within and across social and economic identities to challenge power, privilege, and oppression in support of social and economic justice. This research agenda has been developed through and is grounded in her practice experience, which has focused on community organizing, organizational transformation and leadership, and participatory action research. She utilizes both the breadth and depth of her theoretical and research training to address these intersecting issues with a variety of research methodologies. Her current research focuses on organizing with two constituencies: people with power and privilege, particularly people with wealth, and lesbian, gay, transgender, bisexual, queer, questioning, and allied youth.

Adrienne Dessel, PhD, LMSW is an associate director of the Program on Intergroup Relations (IGR) and Lecturer in the School of Social Work at the University of Michigan. She has over 20 years of experience providing clinical and community based services to diverse client populations and organizations and has worked with school systems in Massachusetts, Pennsylvania, Tennessee, and Michigan. Her community consultations include social justice education for public school teachers and evaluation of LGBT education services. Adrienne teaches courses on intergroup dialogue facilitation, the social psychology of prejudice and intergroup relations, and global conflict and coexistence. Her research focuses on intergroup dialogue processes and outcomes on topics of Arab/Jewish conflict, religion and sexual orientation, gender, and dialogue facilitator learning. Her forthcoming edited book with Dr. Rebecca Bolen is *Conservative Christian Beliefs and Sexual Orientation In Social Work: Privilege, Oppression, and the Pursuit of Human Rights.*

Alex Kulick is a recent graduate of the University of Michigan in women's studies. He has been working with *Riot Youth* at the Neutral Zone in Ann Arbor since he was a teen facilitator and organizer and has been serving as a research collaborator and adult advisor to the program. He also works at the University of Michigan School of Public Health managing the Detroit Youth Passages project, which is a community-based research project examining the relationships between sexual vulnerability, residential instability, and livelihoods among marginalized youth communities in Detroit (www.detroityouthpassages.org). His interests focus on the relationships between intersecting identities, social movements and social change work, and the constructions/performances of diverse gender and sexual identities. He will begin his graduate studies in sociology in the fall of 2014.

Louis F. Graham, DrPH, MPH is an assistant professor in Community Health Education at the University of Massachusetts Amherst School of Public Health with a joint appointment in the Commonwealth Honors College. Using community-based participatory approaches, his scholarship aims to address psychosocial determinants of mental and sexual health among ethnic, gender, and sexually marginalized groups including black and Latino gay and bisexual men and transgender women. Drawing on critical race and queer theories, his current work focuses on structural and institutional factors influencing suicidality and HIV infection among black gay and similarly identified men. He is co-principal investigator of the Detroit Youth Passages project and is a Visiting Professor in the Center for AIDS Prevention Studies at the University of California San Francisco. He also works with community-based organizations to lead evaluation, intervention development, and capacity-building efforts centered on sexual health promotion and protection.

Chapter 1: Introduction: Art in Practice

Jill M. Chonody

"This is MY picture! I'm going to show everyone. Then I'm going to sell it on Ebay!" These were the words of an adolescent that I met during a summer program for youth. As she exclaimed these words to me, it was the first time in more than six weeks that I had seen her light up in quite this way. It was easy to see how proud she was of the image that she created as she showed it off to the other participants in the program along with the staff and her family. This exhibition of work created a unique opportunity for her to showcase her thoughts and feelings, and for her to see those efforts appreciated by her peers and adults alike. This experience of art and empowerment made me want to write to this book. Creative activities are often overlooked in practice, and I believe it is to the detriment of the individuals and groups for whom we engage. Creativity is a shared human potential, and the main aim of this book is to explore how it is something that everyone can incorporate into practice.

There is a separation of art from day to day life. For most of us, we think it is something that other people do. But as children, we did not think much about creativity or self-expression; it was just something that we did. We drew. We painted. We danced. We sang. Yet as our brain develops and matures, our analytical thinking becomes more refined, and we start to look at our art with a critical eye. We judge our work and, for most of us, deem it unworthy. But the creative act itself can be deeply rewarding and source of enjoyment. In fact, creativity is an integral aspect to life, and a capacity that we all possess. Its form may differ and its expression may run the gamut from amateur to professional, but it is the act of creating that is important. Images and other forms of artistic expression can access the human psyche in a way that creates an experience rich with depth and the power to consider life in new ways.

Even if you do not necessarily view yourself as "creative," behaviors to the contrary abound—modifying a recipe, dancing in your living room to your favorite song, making a flower arrangement, or keeping a beautiful garden. This engagement of our imagination is likely to be employed in a multitude of ways each day. Yet, we often do not notice those facets of our imagination as a form of creative expression. But these activities all serve as forms of self-expression and represent who we are as an individual—they are reflections of self. Artistic endeavors incorporate this symbolism in much the same way. We seek to represent our internal, emotional world or abstract concepts and complex experiences in a way that words alone may be lacking. The symbolic environment, including language and representations of culture, provides a way to "communicate…and organize the world" (Ruby, 1981, p. 20).

The creation of art within the context of a therapeutic process or for the expressed purpose to shed light on social conditions allows the viewer to enter into the subjective and symbolic world of the creator. The creation of these abstractions allow for an exploration that supersedes language and verbalizations and taps into something deeper. The use of art is a way to help participants develop their imagination and express their thoughts and feelings. In fact, "visual expression…can do much to precipitate catharsis and reduce internal conflict" (Synder, 1997, p.74). Creative activities are related to positive outcomes for personal well-being and are also linked to healthy aging. If we continue to engage our imagination and the creative aspects of our mind as we age, then we may facilitate life long learning and the maintenance of a healthy brain.

Moreover, community organizing and social change efforts can benefit from the incorporation of creative activities and the production of art. Community building through art is one avenue for meeting goals whether it is engaging residents to assess and create opportunities for change through creative enterprises and outlets, increasing public awareness about social issues, influencing key stakeholders by visually representing community assets and concerns, or developing space within the community for creative expression. Change at the local level can help further build capacity and social capital. For example, photography has been utilized to influence policy in the United Kingdom. A group of people with visual impairment took photographs to illustrate how changes to the busing system could increase their independence. Their images were self-published along with text and then sent to people in positions of power to influence policy (Photovoice, 2013). Artistic techniques and creative enterprises are adaptable to different goals and groups, but matching these prior to undertaking the work is an important first step.

At the heart of artistic efforts in practice is empowerment—an approach that seeks to elevate the voices of those with whom we work. They are the authors of their own lives and thus their voice should be privileged in the process (Rappaport, 1995). Personal narratives are quintessential to who we are, because they are the stories that we tell. They may be personal in nature or reflections of culture, community, and social context, but ultimately they "create memory, meaning, and identity" and are "powerful resources for personal and social change" (Rappaport, 1998, p. 225). Whether working with an individual, group, or community, it is important to start by trying to understand the context. As practitioners[1]—regardless of the level of intervention—we must start where the

---

[1] The term practitioner is being used throughout the book to refer the individual who is organizing the efforts of a particular program, practice or endeavor. It is not meant to isolate community organizers or organizations that may incorporate artistic activities into their work. Similarly, the term participant is being used in a generic way to refer to the people that we work with—which could be a group of people, a whole community, or even the larger society. The term client is used when discussing applications that may occur

individual is. To force our perspective, goals, and needs on others would not lead to change nor would the process leave anyone feeling empowered. For meaningful change to occur, those involved must guide the process, set the goals, and influence the methods that are utilized.

The use of art in practice has a long tradition and takes many forms—drama therapy, expressive arts therapy, creative arts therapy, and music therapy, amongst others. While different theoretical groundings undergird various approaches, the focus of this book is not on those aspects of application. Rather, this book is meant to lay out the literature base for using particular types of creative activities and to give an overview of the evidence that exists to support its use. Practitioners from a variety of disciplines can find use in this book as it does not attempt to counter the professional perspective that comes from creative arts therapy, social work, nursing and the like. This book provides a practical starting point for practitioners from all theoretical and professional backgrounds who would like to incorporate art into their practice.

Organization of This Book

This book has been organized by a particular creative approach, and each of these chapters includes some common elements. Details regarding the use of that approach are explored within the framework of how different groups may benefit from its application. To illustrate one aspect of that technique, an example from the field is offered. Benefits and potential challenges of the approach are provided along with some tips for the practitioner to consider prior to and during implementation. Lastly, a recommended reading list, including helpful websites, is suggested as additional resources.

Starting with Chapter 2, the use of photography is discussed as one avenue for image making. The creation of visual images can be a transformative experience and allows an individual to explore parts of her/himself that are not readily accessible. Photographers chose their composition through the lens of a camera, but it is no less purposeful than other mediums. Both what is included in an image, as well as what is left out, may have significance for the photographer. And the image has the power to move the viewer—it can move you emotionally, propel you into action, or it can stop you in your tracks. Applications of participatory photography for both practice and research are detailed in this chapter.

Storytelling is a natural way to communicate with others, and from a young age, we tell stories. It is a practice that continues throughout our lives and frames who we are. Narrative theory suggests that identity is shaped and transformed by the stories that we tell and is a mode of making meaning from our experiences. All stories exclude, but the content that *is* included gives a window into the person's values, beliefs, and worldview. In Chapter 7, further description of how personal narratives can be transformative and the art of storytelling are explored

---

specifically within the context of therapeutic context—substance treatment counseling, psychotherapy, or other forms of therapeutic intervention where a trained professional is facilitating the process.

as well as the various contexts where it is used. For example, extensive research supports the use of reminiscence with older adults as a way to integrate and reaffirm their identity and life experiences. A practical application of reminiscence with a modern technological twist is detailed in this chapter.

The use of film is becoming an increasingly popular medium as devices become more accessible, both in terms of cost as well as relative ease of use. Most of us carry a device that has the capacity to either take pictures or video, and as a result, both mediums are exploding and becoming a part of our daily lives. When used as a medium for practice, film provides unique benefits, which combines elements of both photography and storytelling. In Chapter 13, digital storytelling is explored and an overview of its evolving use in a range of different applications.

Drawing has the ability to facilitate the expression of powerful emotions, which are often not easily expressed in a clear or linear fashion. Self-expression is depicted through the representations produced by the materials that the participant choses. The use of line, space, color, and composition are all ways that personal information is transformed from a subjective experience into a concrete object. In Chapter 5, drawing is explored, and the communicative functions are reviewed, in particular the ways in which it can express what cannot be realized in language, for example the complex emotions associated with past physical/sexual abuse.

Sculpture, on the other hand, represents a unique form of creative self-expression, because a solid representation of emotions, which are a conduit for memories and insightful meaning, can be made. Clay molding, in particular, is a powerful way to help people express feelings through a tactile connection as well as to facilitate verbal communication and cathartic release. In Chapter 6, the value of sculpture and working with clay are discussed in the context of the healing that takes place for women who have experienced sexual abuse, domestic violence, and childhood traumas.

Similar to sculpture, found and repurposed objects can offer unique opportunities for self-expression given that new meaning can be attached to commonly found items. These objects can be re-worked to create a symbolic self or be used to communicate an emotional state. In Chapter 11, the use of found objects in practice is reviewed. In particular, the configuration of discarded objects and known items (e.g., Lego) is detailed and how this can be used in practice to facilitate exploration of identity and representation of self. Additionally, sand tray therapy can offer clients the opportunity to represent experiences, memories, and fantasies through repurposed objects, including toys, photographs, and household items amongst others. Private practitioner and psychotherapist Caron Leader provides an overview of sand tray therapy, which can be used as an intervention to achieve therapeutic goals.

Another way that creative expression can be reached is through horticultural therapy, which has been utilized with children, older adults, and people who are incarcerated. Offering both educational as well as therapeutic benefits, horticultural therapy can be a simple way to incorporate creativity into practice that does not necessarily require any artistic skills. In Chapter 10, applications of horticultural therapy are explored, and a way it can be used in practice with older adults who are nursing home residents is advanced.

In Chapter 3, street and mural arts are outlined. Street art typically refers to noncommissioned work in which the artist has complete aesthetic control over the production of the piece, which is created in a public space, sometimes without permission and many times, illegally. However, some cities, such as Adelaide, Australia have given over large areas for both the creation of street art as well as community murals (Adelaide City Council, 2013), which are more planned artistic pieces that are maintained over time and considered off limits for other street artists. Initiatives for street art typically focus on youth and other groups who may be socially marginalized, such as Aboriginal and Torres Strait Islanders. Local stencil artist in Adelaide, Joshua Smith, is interviewed about his work with juveniles. Mural arts projects, on the other hand, have been utilized for a variety of community goals as well as personal goals. In Philadelphia, Pennsylvania, the largest mural arts project in the United States exists and is responsible for the creation of more than 3,000 murals in and around the city. Originally started as an initiative to combat graffiti, the murals now symbolize the city and the project has expanded to include efforts focused on restorative justice by working with current and former residents of juvenile and adult criminal justice facilities as well as behavioral and health initiatives (Mural Arts, 2013). The director of the *Restorative Justice Program* for Mural Arts in Philadelphia, Robyn Buseman, is interviewed along with Sara Ansell, program director for the *Porch Light Program* about their efforts.

Performance arts offer unique benefits given that by their very nature they are structured as a group experience. Theater, singing, music, and dancing all share that element of performance, which may help to boost self-esteem and self-confidence for participants. In Chapter 12, the multiple ways that community theater can engage audiences and propel them to make changes in their local areas are explored. In addition, the personal empowerment that can occur through theatrical production are discussed, and a brief overview of drama therapy is outlined. Singing shares some elements that can be found in theater in that it offers singers an opportunity to express themselves, typically in the presence of others. Choirs and other singing activities can be included in a wide range of services and community activities. For older adults, it has been shown to enhance physical, emotional, and mental well-being. This application as well as others is discussed in Chapter 4. Positive benefits are also associated with the creation of music and like singing, musicians are communicating powerful emotions and messages to their audiences. Music communicates a complexity of personal, social, cultural, and political issues, which connects people in a primal way and has the potential to create transformative experiences for its producer as well as its listener. In Chapter 9, the therapeutic advantages of drumming are highlighted, which includes positive intrapersonal and interpersonal outcomes, such as connectedness with others and personal empowerment. Dancing combines movement, music, and visual performance. In Chapter 8, the value of dance is detailed, especially its use as a way to promote personal exploration and provide cathartic experiences for performers and audience members.

Funding bodies, including the government and philanthropic organizations, are increasingly asking for more evaluation of community efforts aimed at the amelioration of social issues and interpersonal problems. Practitioners from all arenas of practice will need to think about how they will evaluate their efforts and demonstrate their impact. At first glance it seems counterintuitive to think about how creativity and evaluation may fit together when in fact, simple evaluative methods of program goals can be used to demonstrate the usefulness of a project. Alternatively, the art itself may be used as a type of data that either illustrates program goals or is a part of a program evaluation. In the final chapter, methods of evaluation are outlined, including quantitative and qualitative approaches to assessment. Also discussed in this chapter is the way in which art may be interpreted. Art may be viewed as both an expression of self as well as a representation of the world around the artist, and issues of interpretation are wrought with potential obstacles. The role of the practitioner, the participant, and the focus of both the project and its evaluation are used to contextualize potential issues associated with interpretation. Wernick and colleagues offer a practical example of how evaluation methods can be used in community programming. *Riot Youth*, which seeks to address bullying, is described, and the evaluators' use of pre/posttest design is explained.

Ethical Issues

In the production of art, many different kinds of ethical issues can arise, including the possibility that strong emotions may surface during the process; something that you may or may not be equipped to handle. This can be addressed by thinking through community resources and appropriate sources for service prior to undertaking such a project. But this is not necessarily something that will occur and depends on the type of project that you are creating. However, one of the most important questions to consider when employing the creation of artistic enterprises in practice is: Who owns this art? Or more specifically, who profits from this work?

Practitioners must be mindful of issues related to ownership and/or copyright. These matters should be discussed up front with participants so there is no confusion regarding who owns their work, how it will be used, and what role its production plays in meeting the goals of the project. For example, if a group of older adults creates a series of photographs that represent their lives in the community as part of a class in the local senior center, then can those photographs be used to promote that particular senior center? Do you need permission from the photographer? What if the images are used to create a calendar, which is then sold to generate money that will support this photography class for other older adults? Are there people depicted in these photographs? And if so, have they given consent for their image to be used? In Chapter 2, these types of issues are discussed when considering ownership of participant generated images. In each of the subsequent chapters, other ethical issues are explored in more detail as they relate to that specific technique.

Audience for This Book

This book is designed for practitioners from a wide variety disciplines, including Social Workers, Psychologists, Community Workers, Nurses, Activities and Recreational Coordinators, Art and Drama Therapists, and Artists and Art Workers. The common element of all these disciplines is the focus on empowerment, change, and self-expression. While some practitioners incorporate creativity by the very nature of their work (e.g., art therapists), they may benefit from exploring the professional examples, tips for application, other fields of creativity, and methods for evaluation. For other disciplines, such as social work, the inclusion of creative or artistic activities are not part of regular practice, but there is no reason it cannot become an essential element. Creative activities align closely with professions that seek to help others. In particular, artistic efforts seek to foster the interpersonal strengths of the participant, which is a general, but common goal amongst such professions as social work, nursing, and recreational therapy.

Similarly, this book is a guide for students majoring in the helping or artistic professions. Those years of study provide a perfect opportunity to explore the ways in which practice can be shaped by creative enterprises and how to challenge the status quo. The addition of creative activities can result in a more inclusive practice for participants—both clients and community members alike— by having the opportunity for expression that supersedes verbal communication. All of this is situated within the contemporary evidence regarding how the approach has been used thus far and how you can evaluate your practice.

The ultimate goal of this book is to help practitioners and future practitioners to think about the ways in which creativity can be merged with their practice— whether you are a community organizer or a person who primarily works with individuals or small groups—creativity can enhance your activities and add depth and meaning. This book guides you in that process and challenges you to think more about how creative you already are. Your creativity can be used to think about new and transformative applications of the artistic expressions detailed here. Combining autobiographical theater and film, storytelling and social media, and photography and social justice are just a few of the combinations that have been explored in these chapters—but the opportunities are limitless. I hope that *Community art: Creative Approaches to Practice* provides a new and exciting learning experience for those already working in the field and those who are just entering it.

References

Adelaide City Council. (2013). *Street art.* Retrieved from http://www.adelaidecitycouncil.com/community/arts-culture/public-art/street-art/#.

Ruby, J. (1981). Seeing through pictures: The anthropology of photography. *Camera Lucida, 3,* 19-32.

Mural Arts. (2013). *Programs: Restorative justice.* Retrieved from http://muralarts.org/programs/restorative-justice.

Rappaport, J. (1995). Empowerment meets narrative: Listening to stories and creating settings. *American Journal of Community Psychology, 23,* 795-807.

Rappaport, J. (1998). The art of social change: Community narratives as resources for individual and collective identity. In X. B. Arriaga & S. Oskamp (Eds), *Addressing community problems: Psychological research and interventions* (pp. 225-246). London: Sage.

Photovoice. (2012). *Sights un*seen. Retrieved from photovoice.org.

Synder, B. (1997). Expressive art therapy techniques: Healing the soul through creativity. *Journal of Humanistic Education & Development, 36,* 74-82.

Chapter 2: Imaging Change: Photography as an Instrument of Practice

Jill M. Chonody & Jill Amitrani-Welsh

"Photographs serve as symbolic images of our human experience and narrow the world as viewed. Persons have the tendency in everyday life to minimize events that create meaning; photography offers a medium to capture everyday events that might otherwise be missed. Later, these events can be revisited through reflection and discussion" (Hagedorn, 1996, p.518).

Introduction

The use of photography in practice or research can be an effective tool in self-expression, communication, and reflection when employed in the manner that best meets the needs of the individual or population. The process of taking photographs allows one to engage with the environment and communicate meaning through those images. Photography has been utilized across many disciplines with a variety of marginalized populations (Weiser, 2013; Stevens & Spears, 2009) and to explore both societal and personal issues (Hagedorn, 1996). It is used for community activism, as a research methodology in anthropology and sociology, and in direct practice. While differences between these methods abound, there is a large overlap in the way that the photographs are employed to achieve particular goals. For most participants, photography is a medium that is relatively easy to use, and they will likely have some level of previous success using it (Weiser, 2004). As technology continues to evolve, picture taking through mobile phones and image sharing in social media are increasingly more mainstream activities. This familiarity with photography could be a way for practitioners to implement the interests and strengths of the individual in their work together.

This chapter explores how individuals can feel empowered through the incorporation of photography in practice and research, including therapeutic benefits associated with the photographic process. We begin with an overview of the ways that photography has been used in research, which includes photo elicitation, participatory photography, and photovoice. Next, we review how these methods have been translated into practice, including a description of phototherapy. Examples from the literature are incorporated to contextualize these methods, including a participatory photography project completed by the authors.

Photo Documentation and Participatory Action Research

Photo documentation is a broad term that encompasses several methods including photo elicitation, participatory photography, and auto photography, just to name a few. While each of these methods operates from a particular research framework, they all make use of photographs in the research process. Photo documentation seeks to empower participants by providing them with the opportunity to record social issues that have meaning to them (Allen, 2012), thus gaining insight into community assets and challenges. Photo documentation is one approach to participatory action research (PAR), which seeks to involve participants in the research process and privileges their perspective. PAR differs from traditional research in that it emphasizes reflection and social action in data collection to improve the well-being of participants and their communities (Baum, MacDougall, & Smith, 2006). We explore how photo elicitation and participatory photography are used in research and then discuss another more structured technique called photovoice.

Photo Elicitation

Photo elicitation is an interviewing technique that uses photographs as a tool for communication to achieve further depth in questioning. The method is an effective way to gather information and create an empowering environment whereby the interviewee is able to explore issues that may not have otherwise been discovered through more traditional methodologies (Clark-IbáÑez, 2004; Hagedorn, 1996). Photo elicitation is typically used as an approach to collecting qualitative data, but using photographs for an in-depth exploration is a common way of using photography in practice. Interviewees can teach the practitioner about their social environment through images, which creates an empowering experience because they are treated as experts. And this is in fact the case—they are the ones who know the most about their lives.

For children, photographs can serve as a concrete prompt (Clark-IbáÑez, 2004). Children can struggle with the interviewing process since it is typically structured around verbal responses to a host of questions. Their attention span may wane, they may not know how to answer certain questions, and they may not have the cognitive capacity to explore a complex topic in this fashion. The use of photographs can bypass these issues and allow for an engaged, creative process to develop. Interpersonal benefits are readily apparent, and this technique has been integrated into various professional practices. In mental health nursing, photographs can be used to guide discussions that help patients tell their story. These discussions can help accentuate the humanizing elements of their condition. Nurses then gain a better understanding of the experiences of their patients. Moreover, using the interviewee's pictures may make the interview process more comfortable (Clark-IbáÑez, 2004) and presents a mechanism for healing by sharing stories (Hagedorn, 1996). In fact, this method is quite similar to how photographs might be used in therapeutic settings, which is discussed in the *Phototherapy* section.

Participatory Action Research

Participatory action research (PAR) is a collaborative research model where members of the community are co-researchers. The goal of this research method is community empowerment by creating a context for the participants to identify problems in their environment and then seek a remedy via social change efforts (Strand, Marullo, Cutforth, Stoecher, & Donohue, 2003). For example, Wilson et al. (2007) used photography as part of an afterschool program whereby students captured challenges within the school and then developed an action plan. One picture depicted a "scary place," an old shed, which students initially wanted to tear down. After learning more about the building and surveying other students' opinions, they decided to make a request to the school district to have the shed painted and made "less scary," which was accomplished.

The use of photography in research with children has allowed their perspectives to be expressed in a way that may not be achieved through more conventional mediums. Photographs can provide insight into what the child finds meaningful as well as allows the researcher to talk to the child about abstract concepts (Cook & Hess, 2007). For example, Aiken and Wingate (1993) engaged three groups of children—those from the "middle-class," children who are homeless, and children with cerebral palsy—to explore ways that they interact with their environment. The children were asked to go on a "photojourney" by taking photographs that represented how they see themselves. Researchers or practitioners who may have previously relied on information from teachers, parents, and siblings can use photography to learn directly from the child. Data gathering through photography enables the communication of everyday experience, thoughts, and feelings without the barriers that may be created by limited cognitive, reading, and oral skills (Dyches, Chichella, Olsen, & Mandleco, 2004). Participants are "encouraged to visually document their social landscapes through photography and reflect on their photographs to produce personal narratives" (Allen, 2012, p. 443). Many writers note that this process can be especially empowering for those groups of people who have been socially marginalized.

PAR highlights how photography can help practitioners learn about their clients and enhance their field of practice. Clients are the best voice for their experience. While this statement seems quite obvious, it can sometimes be missed in a desire to help. By entering into a client interaction with openness and wonder, practitioners can learn about her/his worldview, personal narrative, and social interactions. This can be a way to better understand how a particular issue is experienced and the array of coping skills and resources used to manage it. Furthermore, employing techniques shown to enrich work with clients improves practice and creates greater opportunities for intervention, support, and change.

Photovoice

Photovoice is a more structured approach to PAR, which uses the photographic process to record, reflect, and communicate significance in participants' lives (Wang & Burris, 1994). The goal is to empower people by supporting critical dialogue in group discussions about personal and communal issues and informing policy makers of social problems (Wang & Burris, 1997). Social action occurs when members of the community give meaning to the image and communicate what is needed for change (Wang & Burris, 1997; Wang, 1999). Interpretation of images may reflect social, cultural, and economic conditions. Photovoice has been used with a wide range of populations, including youth (Chonody, Ferman, Amitrani Welsh, & Martin, 2013; Wilson et al., 2007), older adults with chronic pain (Baker & Wang, 2006), individuals with intellectual disabilities (Jurkowski & Paul-Ward, 2007), and people who are HIV+ (Rhodes, Hergenrather, Wilkin, & Jolly, 2008).

Photovoice is also the name of a charitable organization in London that has a focus on social change through participatory photography. Its mission is to ensure a social environment where everyone has an equal opportunity to speak and be heard. By training participants in documentary photography, they are able to create representations of self and develop advocacy skills. Projects include work with people released from incarceration, sexually exploited children, and HIV+ women in Africa (see photovoice.org for further information). The organization and the research application have a number of overlaps, but the most important one is the focus on the voice of participants through photography.

The social action component of participatory photography should reflect participants' goals. Commonly, images are displayed at photo exhibits and presentations with local officials (Wang, 2006; Duffy, 2011). However, social action in a public forum may not always be appropriate. For example, one project led by the developers of the Photovoice organization worked with young, recently arrived refugees. They explored the stigma that they face as refuges in London. This project created a support network for the youth as well as a chance for self-expression in a safe environment (Photovoice, 2013).

Photography as Therapy

Photography in therapeutic settings can take different forms. The use of photographic images can provide for a factual examination of a person, place, or event, but it also allows for the individual to communicate her/his perspective on what is portrayed (Weiser, 2004). There is no standard method or practice for the integration of photography in therapeutic settings (Steven & Spears, 2009), but it most commonly falls in one of two methodologies: photography used as a tool during therapy (i.e., phototherapy; Weiser, 2004) or photography as therapy (i.e., therapeutic photography; Cosden & Reynolds, 1982; Weiser, 2004).

Phototherapy is the use of photographs during a counseling session (Weiser, 2004), and themes designated for the photo shoots can be a guide for healing (Steven & Spears, 2009). For the client, it can facilitate an exploration of self-representation and reconstruction of personal narratives, which in turn may enhance self-esteem. Photography can allow the practitioner to learn more about the client by viewing snapshots, which will likely illustrate family make-up and dynamics, culture, and roles (Weiser, 2004).

> Like footprints on their lives, personal snapshots show not only where people have come from (emotionally as well as geographically), but also foreshadow where they might next be heading, even when they might not know this consciously yet. Sometimes people find that they have taken a photograph, but don't really understand the reason until much later; sometimes the photograph they well remember somehow looks different once they find it and hold it in their hand (Weiser, 2004, p. 24).

The use of images in phototherapy can be particularly helpful in identifying and expressing feelings and when working with clients who are resistant to counseling. The practitioner should never interpret their client's images; rather, the photographs are a tool for communication and exploration of the client's issues (Weiser, 2004; Stevens & Spears, 2009). There are five techniques used in phototherapy.

1. Images taken by the client or created by the client through the use of magazines, cards, the use of the internet, etc.;
2. Photographs that have been taken by other people of the client;
3. Self-portraits;
4. Family (as defined by the client) albums or a collection of photographs that can be explored together for significance;
5. Photo-projective is a process that is unique to the client in that there is an exploration of the decision to photograph the object, event, etc. and the meaning and emotions related to image (Weiser, 2001, 2013).

Phototherapy techniques are interrelated and can yield the greatest response when creatively combined with one another (Weiser, 2001). The practitioner may ask the client to consider different perspectives of the photograph in an effort to better understand the meaning the client associates with the image. Weiser (2004) has found that personal and familial photographs yield emotional and factual information that would have never been revealed just by asking direct questions.

The practitioner focuses more on the feelings and memories provoked by the image than the contents of the photograph. Phototherapy techniques assist the practitioner in identifying recurring images or themes, patterns in the clients' responses, symbolic or remarkable content, consistencies over a time period, and emotional responses to photographs that clients may not be consciously aware that they are expressing. Moreover, asking clients about photographs of themselves can be a helpful way to gain insight into their value system, beliefs, and personal evaluations, all of which can be useful in understanding how the client will assess the quality of their life (Weiser, 2004). Client interpretation of a photograph may also change over time. It may not be until later that some understanding why this was captured or why an older photograph looks different after rediscovering it. For the practitioner, training in phototherapy techniques help determine which photograph to use and at what time. Every photograph has its limitations and benefits to the therapeutic process, and the practitioner needs to know how to adapt the phototherapy techniques to best serve their respective client population (Weiser, 2004). The techniques of phototherapy are typically empowering, especially when working with multicultural, minority, or special needs populations or clients who present with complex situations (Weiser, 2013; Steven & Spears, 2009).

Therapeutic photography, on the other hand, is the use of photography as an intervention in treatment (Weiser, 2004) and can be adapted to circumstances and available resources. It has been used with helping professionals as an exercise of self-care (Caines, 2008) and with Alzheimer's patients to create scrapbook albums of the past (Mitzen, 2007). The photographic process can assist participants in gaining skills around impulse control, social interaction, self-esteem, and acceptance of both positive and critical feedback (Cosden & Renolds, 1982). Therapeutic photography can occur in a group setting with a facilitator or independently, and both approaches can create intrapersonal benefits for participants (Weiser, 2001). Cosden and Reynolds (1982) suggest that therapeutic photography can also be an effective supplement to therapist facilitated therapy, but clearly point out that this technique should not be used as the sole treatment of emotional disorders. Likewise, Weiser (2004) believes the process of photography could result in emotional consequences that may require the assistance of a trained therapist.

Although there are overlapping similarities of phototherapy and therapeutic photography, such as intended outcomes, there are also significant distinctions. While the effectiveness of a therapist in a client's healing process and proper treatment of mental health issues cannot be underestimated in phototherapy, the photographic process in both methodologies presents an opportunity for the client to develop strength-based skills. Since these methodologies hold that there is no "correct" way to interpret a photograph, clients are likely to gain feelings of empowerment and self-awareness, which may be especially true for clients struggling with feelings of self-doubt (Weiser, 2001). However, a clear distinction between these methods is related to the practitioner. Phototherapy requires the involvement of a trained therapist who facilitates a photographic process, which is intended to assist clients in achieving their therapeutic goals. On the other hand, therapeutic photography may include a facilitator, but the focus is more on fostering personal growth. In fact, many therapists trained in phototherapy techniques will also facilitate therapeutic photography groups to provide a more comprehensive counseling experience (Weiser, 2001). In sum, the use of photography to create a context for personal growth and well-being is supported in the literature and may be incorporated into a variety of programs designed for individuals and groups.

Exploring the Images

The images produced by participants/clients will be discussed in some fashion, and the structure used to do so will be shaped by program goals. While there are multiple frameworks available, we introduce two here along with some general suggestions.

It is important to remember that what photographers choose to capture will be reflective of their respective personal and cultural beliefs (Weiser, 2001).

Using open-ended questions when exploring meaning will allow clients to more freely express emotions or perceptions associated with the image (Stevens & Spears, 2009). In phototherapy, Weiser (2004) suggests using less intrusive questions in the beginning, such as:

> What is the story of this photo?
> How did it come to be taken?
> Does it hold any special significance for you, and if so, what?
> What other things (thoughts, memories, feelings) come to mind when you view it? (p. 36-37).

When working with clients in a therapeutic context, it is important to receive the proper training to facilitate both the session as well as the use of photography. The above questions are useful in that context, but could be modified for group work, particularly the question "What is the story of this photo?," which is an open invitation for dialogue. When working with a community group, a broad prompt is useful for initiating a conversation within the group and can facilitate lively discussions of social issues and solutions.

Open-ended questions are also utilized in the reflection component of PAR. Photovoice uses the SHOWeD method for both individual and group processing of images:

1) What do you **S**ee here?
2) What is really **H**appening here?
3) How does this relate to **O**ur lives?
4) **W**hy does this problem or strength exist?
5) What can we **D**o about this? (Wallerstein, 1987).

The practitioner must remember that the participant's emotional response to the photograph cannot be predicted and what is seen in the image will be diferent for every viewer, including the practitioner. Likewise, no singular response to a photograph can fully capture an individual's life (Weiser, 2004). The image represents one facet of that individual and should be explored from that position. Similarly, one image does fully represent a participant's perspective on a particular social issue—the image is one detail in the larger scheme of things. Furthermore, image quality (e.g., composition, lighting, etc) is not typically the main impetus for using photography in practice and should be treated as such. For some participants, constructive criticism of quality may be deterimental to their self-confidence, thus countering your goals.

Case Example: Enhancing Education Goals: Participatory Photography in Action

This participatory photography project was based at an American high school that utilizes project-based learning as a way to facilitate completion of the requirements for a diploma. Students here have had past struggles in traditional school settings, and this alternative high school attempts to re-engage them in their education. The goal of our project was to improve critical thinking through the creation of images from the neighborhood around the school, and the focus of the photographic work was on assets and concerns in the community. A small group of youth (aged 15–18) participated in the project, and all of the students were from the same classroom. The team met with them twice a week over the course of 10 weeks, and each session was approximately two-and-a-half hours. Group photo shoots occurred at the high school, and the second session, held at the university, was structured around group activities and a discussion of their images.

The project team included three members who are trained social workers and one media specialist. The classroom teacher also provided support, guidance, and further structure to the project. In addition to photography, which was the primary medium, we included interactive, educational activities to stimulate their thinking and inform their creation of images. To build rapport, we used various icebreakers and games. For example, we modified a common game where participants are asked to pick between one of two items (e.g., soft drinks, foods, sports teams, etc.). To make the game more relevant, we chose foods, teams, and locations that were representative of the city. They seemed engaged in the game and were willing to verbalize why their choice was the best one, which helped them become more comfortable voicing what matters to them. Once rapport was built within the group, we used other types of activities to facilitate our goals. For example, one exercise was centered on storytelling through the use of images from various magazines. Sitting in a circle, students were asked to look at images placed on the floor and then tell a story, beginning with one picture and then incorporating details using the other images. This exercise was constructive in that students became familiar with the idea that every image has a story.

A number of interesting community concerns were raised by the students, including issues around abandoned buildings, trash, and graffiti. The photo-discussions also stimulated conversation about change. Specifically, they explored how lack of jobs, lack of community outlets, and general disregard contribute to local problems. Students then used their images to produce a final capstone project for their course, which supported larger research projects that they were completing.

A couple of photographs from the project are included here, but it should be noted that these were not taken by the youth. The project team did not seek copyright allowance from participants, and therefore, their images are not included. Nonetheless, these images are representative of the types of photographs that were produced during the project and were taken by a team member, who accompanied students on all of the photo shoots.

The project enjoyed many successes and trials, but the team finished the project feeling that photography can generate conversation and add depth to learning goals. On our last day together, we presented a small gift, a collage of their photographic work, to the students. It seemed as though they felt a sense of accomplishment when we gave them this gift. Perhaps they saw the process as interconnected rather than just individual photo shoots and discussions. To read further reflection on the project by the social work team, please see: Chonody, J. M., Martin, T., & Amitrani Welsh, J. (2014). Looking through the lens of urban teenagers: Reflections on participatory photography in an alternative high school. *Reflections: Narratives of Professional Helping, 18,* 35-44.

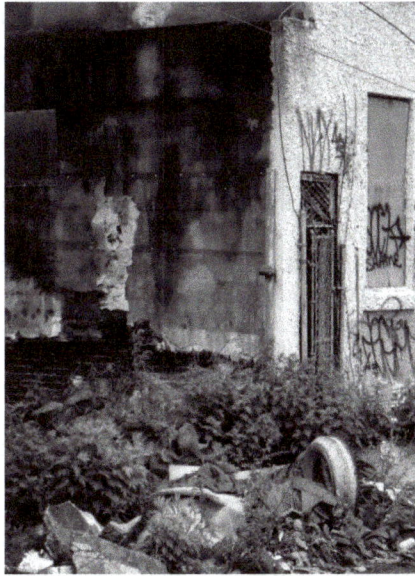

Title: *Trash and an Abandoned Building.*
Location: Philadelphia, PA.
Photo by: Jill Chonody.

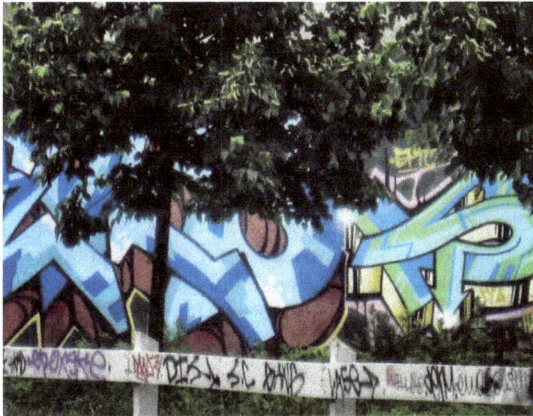

Title: *Graffiti and Tags.*
Location: Philadelphia, PA.
Photo by: Jill Chonody.

Benefits and Potential Challenges

The inclusion of photography in practice has the ability to engage participants in a way that differs from more conventional methods; however, special considerations must also be made. Being aware of the unique dimensions of photography is the best way to prevent potential challenges. In this section, we provide a brief summary of the benefits and limitations of using photography.

The primary benefit of using photography in practice is that it is an inclusive approach to working with various populations, abilities, and social contexts.

When images are viewed collectively, the participant's narrative of her/his history may be visually illustrated and may extend to include a vision of her/his future (Weiser, 2013). These benefits of phototherapy were illustrated in a 12-week outpatient treatment group for adults with chemical dependence. The photographs provided group members with a nonverbal alternative to communication in the initial stages of group work. The image was the starting point in telling their story and provided a structure for the sensitive issues related to their chemical dependency, which were more easily disclosed (Glover-Graf & Miller, 2006).

The use of photography in practice can yield intrapersonal benefits as well as social change. Research involving youth has found that photography is a means to greater development of personal empowerment and involvement in social advocacy and policy reform. Photography projects have helped to increase youth's creativity, writing, reading, and documentary skills (Nolan-Abrahamian, 2009). Despite the benefits of skill development, young people may not outwardly express how they feel about their work during the process, but may be able to explore that aspect later. For example, Allen (2012) found that only after photo elicitation interviews did the young male participants in his project, which was focused on the perspectives of black middle-class youth, exhibit enthusiasm over sharing their experiences and a hopefulness that their work could result in a greater understanding between the youth and school administrators. For others, empowerment may be a process that emerges slowly. For example, Duffy (2011) found that single mothers participating in his photovoice project reported feelings of personal empowerment, an outcome that they had not gained through other therapeutic groups, but it did not happen quickly.

> This concept of "voice" as an important aspect of empowerment developed gradually. Finding their voice and being heard appears to have moved them from helplessness to action. Some participants noted their families or intimate partners never listened to them, and certainly they were not seen or heard in the public/political arena. It is compelling that often lifelong and very negative messages could be altered over a 2-year period through a relational interactive process that offers a safe, respectful, and nonjudgmental space (Duffy, 2011, p. 111).

A year and a half after the photovoice project, four of the women were still meeting to maintain their relationships and the support system they had created (Duffy, 2011). The benefits of photography in practice and research may vary and may not always be evident throughout the process, especially for those participants who may take longer to realize that the importance of their perspective. But for some, the use of photography offers life-altering changes, including the development of support networks and improved self-confidence.

Unique barriers to participation relative to the population may also need to be considered when implementing a photography project. Complex life circumstances may preclude full participation. For example, in Duffy's (2011) study with single mothers, personal challenges with employment, chronic health conditions, depression, and child-care often prevented some women from participating. Considering issues such as these before starting a project will allow for contingency plans and help prepare the practitioner for feelings of disappointment or frustration that may occur in response to these issues. When working with individuals with developmental disabilities or other cognitive incapacities, further considerations may need to be made. For example, participants may experience difficulty articulating their thoughts in written form or reading and completing surveys or questionnaires and may need additional technology to effectively use the camera (Finlay & Lyons, 2001; Dyches et al., 2004). The approach is adaptable to these needs, but they should be thoughtfully considered up front.

A final challenge to consider when using photography in practice is issues of censoring. This can occur if parents limit their children by forbidding them to take the camera outside the home or set rigid parameters on what they are allowed to photograph. This may also occur if a project is taking place within an institutional setting where residents may have limited capacity. Similarly, censorship can occur when images are deleted from a digital camera or prints are removed prior to meeting back with the practitioner. This could be relevant in a variety of contexts. If the practitioner is collecting data as part of a project, then censorship limits the data and perhaps biases the process. In practice, censorship could actually provide insights into family dynamics or other issues that the participant may be facing, such as a controlling partner. In either scenario, the practitioner should be mindful of the context that her/his participants originate as this may provide clues as to why there are no pictures or missing pictures. It would be easy to jump to the conclusion that the participant just decided not to do the assignment for the week, when in fact, more complex issues may be at work.

Photography provides distinctive benefits as well as challenges to practitioners and participants. One of the standout features of photography is that "cognitive, linguistic, and motor demands are minimal, as the photographer primarily uses visual skills to distinguish the subject of the photograph" (Dyches et al., 2004, p.174). Spending time up front to think about potential issues will have a huge pay off once the project/program begins.

Ethical Considerations

Considering that photography is a tool for change, understanding ethical considerations can help provide the best care for participants. Visual media introduces additional responsibilities, and the following discussion is inclusive of different types of practice using photography, which should be considered during the planning stages of a project.

When working with a group, whether it is for the purposes of research, community development, or personal enrichment, the practitioner will need to decide if cameras will be supplied to participants. Ethical dilemmas may arise when participants are responsible for financial compensation of a lost/damaged camera, particularly if the participant has an unstable financial situation (Allen, 2012). Similarly, if cameras are supplied to participants for the purposes of completing the project, then are they expected to return them when it is finished? Practitioners will need to create a balance between financial constraints from funders or shrinking organizational budgets and the consequences associated with providing an opportunity and activity for people who may be marginalized and then abruptly removing it. These dilemmas should be resolved prior to the project and discussed with participants at initial meetings.

Likewise, determining ownership and rights of use for images created during a project should be discussed with participants upfront (Weiser, 1986). Phototherapy and photo elicitation for purposes of therapeutic intervention or interviewing does not create the same types of dilemmas that would be found when working in community projects or other group contexts. For therapeutic purposes, the clients would bring snapshots with them to be used in the office. Issues of ownership should not arise when photographs are limited to this narrow scope. However, when working with groups, copyright and image use is a major concern. An open conversation with participants about expectations maintains the focus on empowerment. Some practitioners may feel that the right to use images is theirs since they developed and facilitated the project. The key issue here is that the practitioner is not the photographer. For some projects, the need to generate income to support the program is a real necessity; therefore, practitioners may want to sell the images created by participants as prints, cards, books, or calendars. While there is nothing unethical about this per se, participants should have the right to refuse, and the process should be transparent. Participants can be included in the creation of such products and given a portion of the proceeds. For example, photographer Nancy McGirr began working with children in Guatemala City who were living in a dump, and they were given cameras to document their experiences. Later these images, along with their writings, were turned into a book, *Out of the Dumps*. The proceeds are used to fund the children's education. Innovative ways to create beneficial situations for participants are endless; each of these issues just needs to be clearly detailed and openly explored with participants.

A related consideration is rights to privacy. Rights to privacy refer to both public and private spaces. Specifically, participants need to be able to identify when consent is needed to take the photograph of another person, and in turn, how that image may be used later. Ethical issues of representing people from oppressed or vulnerable situations are of particular concern. If the images will be used in some kind of public forum, such as an exhibition, then featuring recognizable faces is not appropriate unless the photographer has received written consent. Similarly, if participants are featured in each other's images, then both the photographer and the subject should give consent before that image is used for any other purpose. Issues of participant safety are also related to consent given that some community participatory photography projects take place in areas that may have significant social issues, which can put participants at risk.

Finally, the practitioner should explore the context of the method, its focus, and the respective population prior to beginning the work. For example, how will the method be empowering for participants? What is the main focus for this work? The expectations communicated to participants about possible outcomes should always be realistic and attainable (Strand et al., 2003). Information regarding the process and its intention should be presented in a manner that can be understood by all perspective participants, particularly when working with individuals who have cognitive or intellectual disabilities. Should there be questions about an individual's ability to comprehend the purpose or the implications of their involvement in the research process, then parents or guardians should be included (Boxall & Ralph, 2009). When using photography in practice, practitioners should also consider issues of capacity, but if the images are used for personal exploration instead of public displays or publishable research reports, then this may be less of an issue.

Other ethical issues related to the creation and exhibition of photographic images could not be included here, but additional resources are offered in the *Recommended Readings and Resources* at the end of this chapter.

Tips for Practitioners

1.   **Who will take the pictures?** Will the practitioner take photographs with participants? For them? Or will participants take pictures and then display the images of their choice? Which approach is consistent with your goals?

2.   **What kind of cameras will you use? Who will provide them?** There are many cameras to choose from—iPhone/smart phone technology, disposable film cameras, digital cameras, SLR, etc. Finding a balance between the amount of photographic training and the degree of direction provided before photo shoots is essential in preparing participants. If there is not a clear understanding of how to use the camera, then participants may experience feelings of embarrassment, and as a result, their perspective will not be adequately captured (Packard, 2008). You may want to consider other factors when making your choice, such as what skill level are your participants? Will you need a professional to give some training? Are there any issues related to dexterity that should be considered for your group (e.g., eyesight, arthritis, mobility, tremors, etc.)? The logistics around the cost of purchasing the cameras, the repayment of lost cameras (Clark-IbáÑez, 2004; Allen, 2012), and the level of accountability participants have for the cameras (Allen, 2012) should be considered. Using low-cost cameras may increase the likelihood that participants of varying abilities could participate (Packard, 2008), but their use may have other implications. For example, some participants may not use a disposable camera because of the perception that it means that they could not afford better technology (Allen, 2012). The logistical issues of organizing the distribution and collection of cameras and the development of film may also be too costly and time constraining (Clark-IbáÑez, 2004). If cameras are provided, can they be gifted to participants if the project has a natural completion date?

3.   **What is the goal for the use of photography? What is the end product of your project?** Do you hope to elicit change in the community? How will you accomplish that goal (e.g., exhibits with key stake holders) and then how will you assess it? Do you hope to raise money for a cause? Would you like to produce a specific product to be used to sustain the project? Have you discussed your ideas with participants?

4.   **What are your expectations for the images?** Have you thought about the wide range of image quality that participants will create? Can you

work with almost any image quality that the participant produces? Are you secretly hoping that the photographs will be of museum quality?

5. **What are your plans for processing images with participants?** What methods will you use to explore the images that participants create? A standardized framework? Will you suggest possible interpretations and underlying symbolism to your participants? What consequences might be anticipated as the result of your choice?

6. **How will you build rapport with your participants and communicate your goals?** Participatory photography will not be an empowering experience if participants do not believe that their insights matter (Packard, 2008; Allen, 2012). The practitioner will want to build rapport and may need work with participants on valuing their voice before implementing the photo shoots. If you are working with a group of people, who will likely have their own perspectives and preferences for how to accomplish the goals of the group, how will you build cohesiveness? How much direction will you give for photo assignments? Insufficient information regarding theme(s) of the photo shoot(s) could lead to anxiety or feelings of inadequacy to successfully complete the assignment. As a result, the photo shoot could be limited with very few to no pictures taken. On the other hand, too much direction stifles creativity. Either way, this type of experience has the potential to abate the empowering impact of the process for the individual.

7. **How will you address issues of safety?** Phrases like "be safe" or "be smart" without expanding on what good decision-making looks like in photography should be avoided. This is especially critical when working with youth or individuals with limited intellectual capacity, and additional steps to ensure safety should be made. For example, a role-play can be used to process potential safety issues. By working through common situations that participants could face, they will feel more comfortable if in fact they find themselves in that situation. This approach works particularly well when working with a group as they can brainstorm the situations; however, the process can be modified and accomplished as a one-on-one activity.

8. **Have you thought about how to manage issues of time?** Photography takes time. Participants will need time to take photographs, explore related topics, perhaps complete a written activity, and the space to think about meaning. Projects also need time for fun. Can you incorporate activities that are purely for the joy of the experience, such as photo shoot scavenger hunt?

9. **Do you need institutional support before implementing a photography project?** Certain agencies and organizations, such as prisons and nursing homes, have significant reservations about allowing people to have access to cameras. Not only can it pose an issue of safety, but it also presents issues surrounding privilege and exposure that administrators are reticent to allow. In some cases, this can be overcome, but it is worth thinking about as you plan your project.

10. **Have you matched your program activities to the needs, wants, and abilities of your group?** Issues of literacy, dexterity/mobility, cognitive

abilities, and physical capabilities are amongst the things that should be explored when planning various activities that are to be accomplished. This is not limited to just taking pictures, but other tasks that you will do as part of your overall plan to achieve your goals.

Recommended Readings and Resources

Ballerini, J. (1997). Photography as a charitable weapon: Poor kids and self-representation. *Radical History Review, 69,* 160-188.

Dragan, P. B. (2008). *Kids, cameras, and the curriculum: Focusing on learning in the primary grades.* Portsmouth, NH: Heinemann.

Ewald, W. (2001). *I wanna take me a picture: Teaching photography and writing to children.* Boston, MA: Beacon.

Gross, L., Katz, J. S., & Ruby, J. (Eds.). (1988). *Image ethics: The moral rights of subjects in photographs, film, and television.* Oxford: Oxford University Press.

Photovoice. (2013). *Free online resources.* Available at: photovoice.org/shop/info/methodology-series.

Photovoice Manual. (2013). *From snapshot to civic action: A photovoice facilitator's manual.* Available at: http://ces4health.info/uploads/from%20Snapshot%20to%20Civic%20Action~%20A%20Photovoice%20Facilitator%E2%80%99s%20Manual.pdf.

Riley, G., & Manias, E. (2004). The uses of photography in clinical nursing practice and research: A literature review. *Journal of Advanced Nursing, 48,* 397-405.

Weiser, J. (1999). *PhotoTherapy techniques: Exploring the secrets of personal snapshots and family albums.* Vancouver, B.C.: PhotoTherapy Centre.

References

Aitken, S. C., & Wingate, J. (1993). A preliminary study of self-directed photography of middle-class, homeless, and mobility-impaired children. *Self-Directed Photography, 45*(1), 65-72.

Allen, Q. (2012). Photographs and stories: Ethics, benefits and dilemmas of using participant photography with black middle-class male youth. *Qualitative Research, 12*(4), 443-458.

Baker, T., & Wang, C. (2006). Photovoice: Use of a participatory action research method to explore the chronic pain experience in older adults. *Qualitative Health Research, 16*(10), 1405-1413.

Baum, F., MacDougall, C., & Smith, D. (2006). Participatory action research. *Journal of Epidemiology & Community Health, 60,* 854-857.

Boxall, K., & Ralph, S. (2009). Research ethics and the use of visual images in research with people with intellectual disability. *Journal of Intellectual & Developmental Disability, 34*(1), 45-54.

Caines, J. (2008). The picture of health: A heuristic self-inquiry of therapeutic photography as self-care for helping professions. Retrieved from https://www.uleth.ca/dspace/bitstream/handle/10133/789/caines,%20jana-lynn.pdf?sequence=1.

Chonody, J. M., Ferman, B., Amitrani-Welsh, J., & Martin, T. (2013). Violence through the eyes of youth: A photovoice exploration. *Journal of Community Psychology, 41,* 84-101.

Clark-IbáÑez, M. (2004). Framing the social world with photo-elicitation interviews. *American Behavioral Scientist, 47*(12), 1507-1527.

Cook, T., & Hess,T. (2007). What the camera sees and from whose perspective: Fun methodologies for engaging children and enlightening adults. *Childhood, 14*(1), 29-45.

Cosden, C., & Reynolds, D. (1982). Photography as therapy. *The Arts in Psychotherapy, 9,* 19-23.

Duffy, L. (2011). "Step-by-step we are stronger": Women's empowerment through photovoice. *Journal of Community Health Nursing, 28,* 105–116.

Dyches, T. T., Cichella, E., Frost, S. O., Mandleco, B. (2004). Snapshots of life: Perspectives of school-aged individuals with developmental disabilities. *Research & Practice for Persons with Severe Disabilities, 29*(3), 172-182.

Finlay, W. M., & Lyons, E. (2001). Methodological issues in interviewing and using self-report questionnaires with people with mental retardation. *Psychological Assessment, 13*(3), 319-335.

Franklin, K. L., & McGirr, N. (Eds). (1995). *Out of the dump: Writings and photographs by children from Guatemala.* New York: Lothrop, Lee & Shepard Books.

Glover-Graf, N., & Miller, E. (2006). The use of phototherapy in group treatment for persons who are chemically dependent. *Rehabilitation Counseling Bulletin, 49*(3), 166-181.

Hagedorn, M. I. E. (1996). Photography an aesthetic technique for nursing inquiry. *Issues in Mental Health Nursing, 17,* 517-527.

Jurkowski, J., & Paul-Ward, A. (2007). Photovoice with vulnerable populations: Addressing disparities in health promotion among people with intellectual disabilities. *Health Promotion Practice, 8,* 358-365.

Mitzen, M. (2007). Scrapbook photo albums are therapeutic for Alzheimer's patients. *Creative Memories.* Retrieved from www.creativememories.com/Alzheimers Album.PDF.

Nolan-Abrahamian, E. (2009). Photography in the field: Empowering youth and affecting public policy. *Youth Media Reporter, 1,* 7-10.

Packard, J. (2008). "I'm gonna show you what it's really like out here": The power and limitation of participatory visual methods. *Visual Studies, 23,* 63-77.

Photovoice. (2013). *Transparency: Living without borders.* Retrieved from http://www.photovoice.org/projects/uk/transparency-living-without-borders.

Rhodes, S. D., Hergenrather, K. C., Wilkin, A. M., & Jolly, C. (2008). Visions and voices: Indigent persons living with HIV in the Southern United States use photovoice to create knowledge, develop partnerships, and take action. *Health Promotion Practice, 9,* 159-169.

Strand, K., Marullo, S., Cutforth, N., Stoecher, R., & Donohue, P. (2003). *Community-based research and higher education.* San Francisco, CA: Jossey-Bass.

Stevens, R., & Spears, E. (2009). Incorporating photography as a therapeutic tool in counseling. *Journal of Creativity in Mental Health, 4,* 3–16.

Wallerstein, N. (1987). Empowerment education: Freire's ideas applied to youth. *Youth Policy, 9,* 11–15.

Wang, C. C. (1999). Photovoice: A participatory action research strategy applied to women's health. *Journal Women's Health, 8,* 185-192.

Wang, C. C. (2006). Youth participation in photovoice as a strategy for community change. *Journal of Community Practice, 14*(1-2), 147-161.

Wang, C. C., & Burris, M. A. (1994). Empowerment through photo novella: Portraits of participation. *Health Education and Behavior, 21,* 171-186.

Wang, C. C., & Burris, M. A. (1997). Photovoice: Concept, methodology, and use for participatory needs assessment. *Health Education and Behavior, 24,* 369- 387.

Weiser, J. (1986). Ethical considerations in phototherapy training and practice. *Phototherapy, 1*(1), 12-17.

Weiser, J. (2001). Phototherapy techniques: Using clients' personal snapshots and family photos as counseling and therapy tools. *Afterimage: The Journal of Media Arts and Cultural Criticism, 29*(3), 10-15.

Weiser, J. (2004). Phototherapy techniques in counselling and therapy—using ordinary snapshots and photo-interactions to help clients heal their lives. *The Canadian Art Therapy Association Journal, 17*(2), 23-56.

Weiser, J. (2013). *Phototherapy techniques in counseling and therapy.* Retrieved from http://www.phototherapy-centre.com/home.htm.

Wilson, N., Dasho, S., Martin, A. C., Wallerstein, N., Wang, C., & Minkler, M. (2007). Engaging young adolescents in social action through photovoice: The Youth Empowerment Strategies (YES!) project. *The Journal of Early Adolescence, 27, 241-261.*

Chapter 3: Painted on the Wall: How Street and Mural Art Can Be Transformative

Jill M. Chonody

The artists and agitators who are decorating our built environment are simultaneously invoking millennia-old art forms, echoing pre-literate and pre-industrial signage and jumping across the chasms of the digital divide and the complete commercialization of public communication (Howze, 2008, p. 6).

Introduction

The use of images to communicate information can be traced back some 20,000 years to cave paintings (Howze, 2008), and in addition to storytelling, these paintings may be thought of as an early form of public art given their role within the social group. In a contemporary context, public art takes many forms—mosaics, fountains, paintings—and the use of art as a form of communication has proliferated. In New York City, for example, the transit system has its own public art program, which includes both permanent and temporary artwork as well as posters and poetry (MTA, 2013). The beautification of the subway system is thought to enhance the daily commute (view their collection here: www.mta.info/mta/aft/about/), and through public display, the importance of art is represented. While all public art has the potential to create an impact for both viewer and artist, the focus of this chapter is exclusively dedicated to public artwork in the form of street and mural art.

Defining Street and Mural Art

Graffiti is a continuum from the unabashedly ugly to the unavoidably beautiful (Gastman, Neelon, & Smyrski, 2007, p. 127).

Street art and graffiti art are often used as interchangeable terms to describe a form of public art, that while still illegal in many places, is easily distinguishable from what most would think of as traditional graffiti or bombing—"the act of getting your name up illegally and irrespective of the pretense of marking 'art'" (Gastman et al., 2007, p. 127). Tags and bombing are likely the most despised form of graffiti and the most abundant, yet even this type of graffiti can take on an art form (see photograph *Tags and Street art* below). Street art, on the other hand, is not just graffiti or just art—rather it is a new kind of visual representation that surpasses both categories. The walls of the city have become the new canvas (Austin, 2010), and street art, which encompasses stencils, stickers, paste-ups (see pictures below), and murals, has emerged from the graffiti movement and moved worldwide. The term "mural" used within the context of street art refers to those large-scale works produced in public spaces that are likely to be unsanctioned by the community and possibly illegal (see *Melbourne Alleyway* for an example).

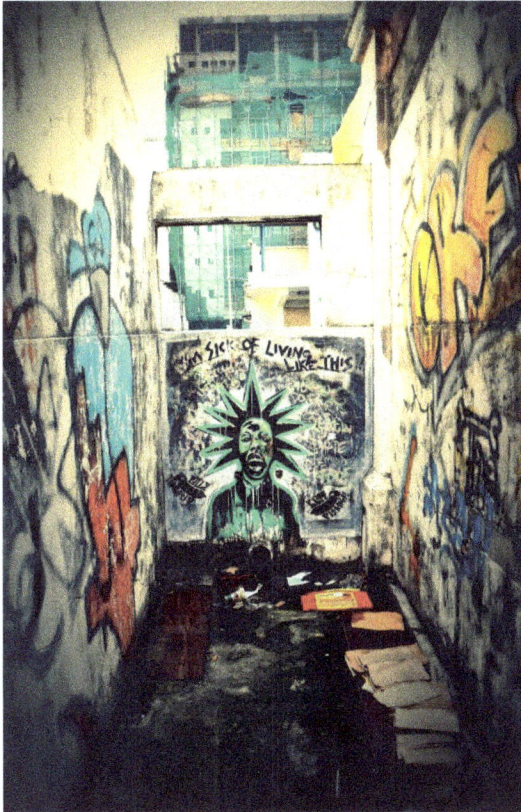

Title: *Tags and Street art.*
Artists: Unknown.
Location: Kota Kinabalu, Malaysia.
Photo by: Jill Chonody.

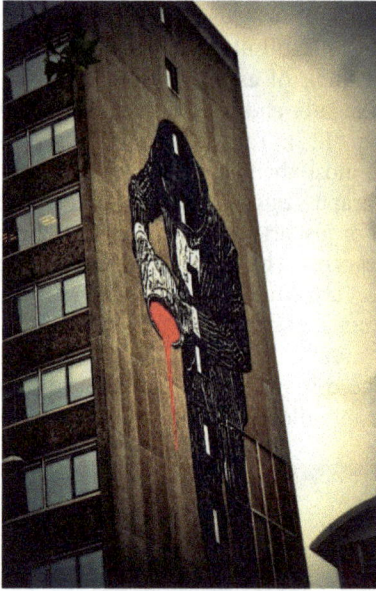

Title: *Stencil*.
Artist: Unknown.
Location: Bristol, U.K.
Photo by: Jill Chonody.

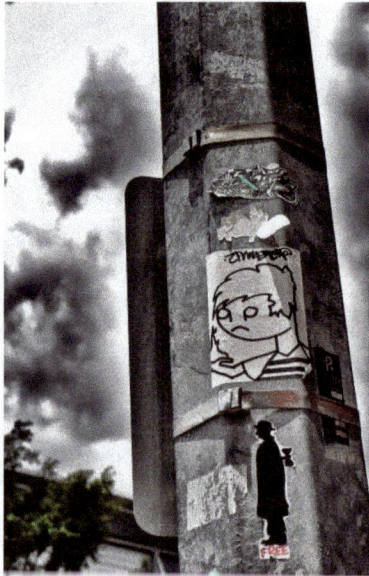

Title: *Stickers*.
Artists: Unknown.
Location: Brisbane, Australia.
Photo by: Jill Chonody.

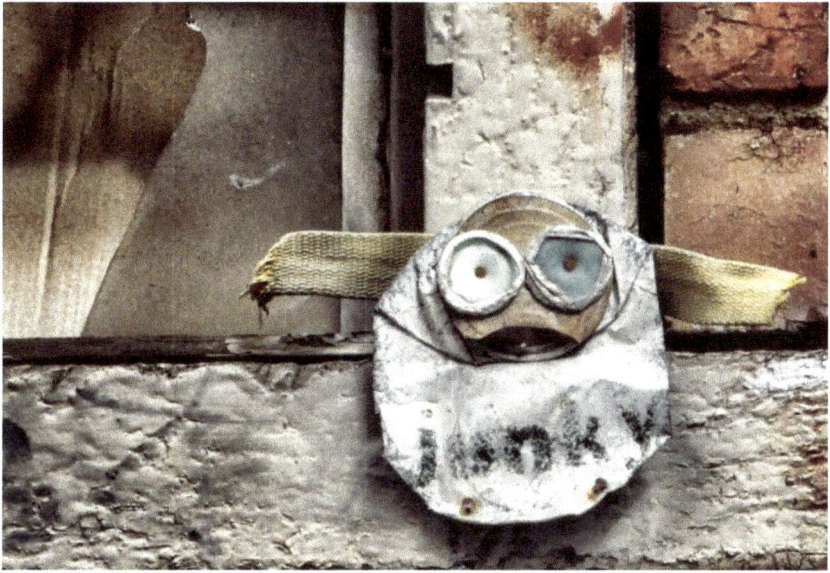

Title: *Three Dimensional Paste-Up*.
Artist: Unknown.
Location: Melbourne, Australia.
Photo by: Jill Chonody.

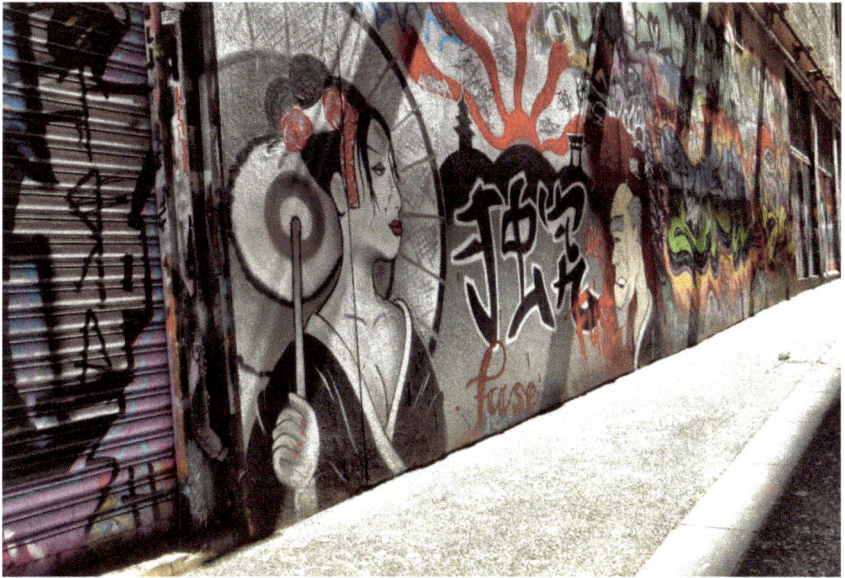

Title: *Melbourne Alleyway*.
Artist: Unknown.
Location: Melbourne, Australia.
Photo by: Jill Chonody.

Street art is "a potential *enhancement* to everyday urban life" (emphasis in the original; Austin, 2010, p. 34) and can be a way to communicate important information via physical spaces (Howze, 2008). A type of "political discourse" or a representation of social problems may be the focus of the art, which can compel both creator and viewer to ask bigger questions (Howze, 2008). For example, the anonymous United Kingdom artist Bansky, probably the best-known street artist, creates stencils that underscore social and political issues, including homelessness and warmongering. He creates murals that support those who are without social power and question oppressive activities by the government (Gastman et al., 2007; for images, see: http://www.banksy.co.uk/). Nonetheless, his work remains an illegal act in most parts of the world.

Alternatively, some cities provide "legal walls" for street art (e.g., Santiago, Barcelona, Paris, and Melbourne amongst others; Gastman et al., 2007), which provide an opportunity to work with others directly in the medium of an open space. Since these walls are "free," space for artists is available to showcase their work or achieve other group goals. Even when legal walls are unavailable, alternatives may still be available for graffiti art. Research in New York City indicates that some street artists are moving into the category of "legal graffiti artists." Through interviews with 20 local street artists, Kramer (2010) found that many of them seek ways to produce legal artwork by approaching small businesses and requesting permission to paint one of their outer walls. Either one person or a group of graffiti artists, up to 20 people in some cases, then produce these works (Kramer, 2010).

To distinguish street art from a more common approach to painting on public walls or spaces, the terms "mural art" and "community mural art" are used. This form of public art is both legal and has the consent of the community. Mural art projects often seeks direct input from community members in their creation. The involvement of local people can be just as important as the mural itself, which is what distinguishes it from commissioned or commercial artwork (Marschall, 2002). Mural arts programs can be found in various cities in the United States, including one such program in Chicago, Illinois, which has a focus on community building through intergenerational projects and youth based programs geared toward art education. Some of the murals created through that initiative can be viewed at: www.cpag.net/home/wwd_latestwork.html.

Public art in its various forms has been utilized to achieve a number of different goals including communication of political/social discontent, representation of the community, a point in history, and as a therapeutic outlet for those who are incarcerated, psychiatrically hospitalized, or socially stigmatized. Nonetheless, very little research exists on how the creation of public art can be used in practice, and most available writings are descriptive in nature. This chapter will bring together this descriptive information along with case examples and the scant research available on this topic to provide an overview of how this creative outlet may be used to produce both individual and community change.

Using Street and Mural Art in Practice

Despite the limited research, mural arts are a fairly common expressive outlet, and generally speaking, are used to: create a sense of community, educate, engage with marginalized groups, and achieve restorative justice or behavioral health goals. Though street art remains illegal in many places, its principles can still be included in other more innovative and lawful ways. It has the potential to be a powerful outlet for working with people, especially youth, and applications would be similar to those of mural arts. Utilizing examples of street art described in the literature, suggestions on how to create legal and realistic projects are offered along with available research and examples on mural arts.

Creating Community and Facilitating Change

Street Art

A straightforward way to include street art in practice would be to incorporate it into a class within a school, community center, or program aimed at vulnerable adolescents. Participants could first view various examples of street art (e.g., Banksy, Shepherd Fairey, etc) and discuss its role in the broader social context. Next, participants could create their own social commentary artwork based on local or personal issues (e.g., violence). Utilizing a wide range of artistic modalities (e.g., spray paint, stencils, stickers), the final products could then be presented in a public forum to initiate further dialogue. Key public figures could be invited to view the pieces and to participate in an exploration about community change. Personal empowerment along with influencing local change would be central benefits of such an approach. Moreover, this would provide a way to document the strengths and history of that community.

Another possibility for groupwork may be a modification of the radical posters that papered the walls of Paris in 1968. This effort sought to educate the public about growing dissatisfaction with the government and "was all at once a political, artistic and informational experiment;" through an image on a poster, the spirit of a movement was communicated (McGrogan, 2008, p. 34). The basic idea of poster distribution could also be translated into a smaller scale change effort. For example, teachers could help students to organize and create their own "poster revolution" for change on an issue that they have identified as essential to their education, community, or health and well-being. Such an effort is indicative of both public art and social justice with the potential to empower students by having their voices heard.

Mural Arts

By their very nature, mural art can facilitate community connections. A sense of ownership and a source of shared experience may be generated by their very existence. For example, Moss (2010) found that local residents in Philadelphia (the "City of Murals") developed a connection with the murals found around the city, particularly the portraits. The murals became a point of reference ("Have you seen Patti [LaBelle] yet?") and "reinforced an imagined sense of community among those who have never actually met" (Moss, 2010, p. 387). Although local residents did not necessarily decide on the specific content of the mural, the murals do seem to reflect community desire. Moreover, in a study in Durban, South Africa, Marschall (1999) found that local residents enjoyed area murals and a "respect for walls or buildings" emerged in that they remained graffiti-free, often for many years (p. 78). This approach to using mural arts requires a skilled artist who is knowledgeable about the community. Additional input from local residents on the content, composition, and location will reinforce connections to it.

The significance of community participation is important to note. In Marschall's (1999) study, residents reported that they did not necessarily feel like the murals were "theirs"—it was something that was added to their neighborhood. Community participation influences the perception of mural art and illustrates the importance of participatory projects. In data collected from two different creative projects—one a mural and the other a play—the role of local residents was found to be fundamental in creating community connection (Hutzel, 2007). Both projects provided residents the opportunity to build new relationships while achieving a common goal. Both also demonstrated how participant driven projects could lead to empowerment, specifically the belief that local change is possible. For example, in this study, young people created murals in an area where violence, trash, and drugs were commonplace, and by reclaiming the area, participants were able to affect immediate aesthetic change (Hutzel, 2007). Organizing within the community to create a mural can be a powerful way for residents to exert power and control in their immediate environment. City walls, abandoned buildings, alleys, and doorways may provide prime spots for beautification and offer an opportunity to work with the community to make these changes. In sum, community based participatory murals highlight how public art can be used to create a sense of connection within and pride in the community.

Education

Street Art

Educational endeavors may be facilitated by the use of street art and other kinds of subversive public art. For example, this type of art could be toured in the local community or images could be viewed in a classroom setting and then used to facilitate discussion about global (or local) social issues and pressing problems. Furthering the conversation and the learning process could be achieved through other activities, such as creating art pieces, writing essays, or researching social issues. This type of approach may be particularly compelling for younger people—from middle school through to university—who may be in touch with these cultural movements.

Similarly, educational projects that make use of modification of existing images and objects may provide another outlet. Street artists sometimes modify objects (e.g., signs) to communicate social protest. In Sydney, Australia, for instance, a group of individuals called BUGA UP (Billboard Utilising Graffitists Against Unhealthy Promotions) began altering billboard advertisements to create new messages. For example, a billboard for Marlboro originally read: "New. Mild. And Marlboro." After modification, it read: "New. Vile. And a bore" (as illustrated in Iveson, 2013, p. 948). Using modification of existing images or the creation of three-dimensional art products from repurposed materials may offer a realistic and legal avenue for engaging youth. For example, the practitioner could use magazine advertisements (such as beauty advertisements) and have participants subject them to modification as a form of social commentary. Allowing participants to determine the focus of the effort will create greater buy-in, and the inclusion of public display will encourage critical thinking. A project like this could be employed at a community center or in a classroom setting at school or even a project displayed to the wider community through a gallery-type forum. Consciousness-raising can occur through public display, and personal empowerment may come from showcasing one's work.

Mural Art

Similar to street art, educational outcomes can also be achieved through mural arts. Across the United States and all over the world, many cities are fortunate to have vast arrays of public art that is available not only for everyone's viewing, but could also become the focus of educational endeavors. By engaging students with community murals, street art, or graffiti, a new opportunity to discuss art and its context are created and a bridge for larger conversations emerges. While this approach is not centered on mural creation, it still represents a way that art can be transformative. For example, in Detroit, artist Tyree Guyton is creating community works of art for the expressed purpose that "it encourages people to talk about difficult issues including politics, racism, religion, poverty, homelessness, and consumption" (Buffington, 2007, p. 26). It is through dialogue that social change can begin to happen. Instructional approaches may help students engage with the art to achieve the goals of:

1. understanding that there are multiple interpretations of and reactions to works of art;
2. discussing how laws affect public works of art;
3. explaining and defending their views of the Heidelberg Project (Guyton's public art initiative, see: http://www.heidelberg.org/);
4. creating works of art using found objects that communicate their ideas about a contemporary subject (Buffington, 2007, p. 26).

For those who do not live in Detroit and have access to such an innovative project, these objectives could be applied in their local community utilizing available public art. Alternatively, if public art is unavailable, the *Resources and Readings* list at the end of the chapter provides some suggestions for books that contain images of various kinds of public art. *Google Images* also offer a plethora of photographs from around the world, which could be used instead.

Mural creation, on the other hand, can be used to integrate multiple forms of knowledge. Student projects aimed at the design and development of a mural have a long history within schools. Fradella (2005) describes such a project where a group of 15 middle school students in an after-school art group were charged with creating an historical mural. Students completed research for the project and then collaborated to determine what images would be included. To determine how best to portray their composition, math was utilized for proportion, scale, and measurement. Reflective writing exercises and dabbling in color theory added the dimensions of language arts and science. Fradella (2005) indicates that these students not only learned concrete matters regarding history, but they learned invaluable life lessons, including cooperative learning, peer education, and joint planning. Moreover, this project helped to increase their self-confidence and social skills. Creating themed murals in schools, community centers, or other public spaces can offer a modality for engaging youth to achieve both educational and personal goals.

Restorative Justice and Prison Rehabilitation

Street Art

Restorative justice principles are based on the idea that the criminal justice system is overly reliant on incarceration, which is detrimental for minor offenses, especially amongst vulnerable youth. As an alternative to jail sentences and probation, community-based sanctions can focus on rehabilitation, reparations to the community, and accountability of actions (Barnard, 2013). The movement toward legal street art may provide an opportunity for collaborative efforts with local agencies, practitioners, or other organizations to achieve restorative justice. For example, practitioners could work with youths who have been caught tagging and seek to approach one of those businesses to create a street art mural as a way to give back. Murals often remain graffiti-free (re: tags), and this approach utilizes restorative justice, urban beautification, and personal empowerment. Moreover, some street artists may be interested in mentoring youth and helping them to develop their skills so that they may pursue avenues of legal artistic production (see *Teaching Street Art: An Example of How a Community Deals with Graffiti* for an example).

Case Example: Teaching Street Art: How a Community Deals with Graffiti

Street artist and gallery owner Joshua Smith spends part of his time teaching workshops for youth in and around Adelaide, South Australia. Joshua has been a graffiti artist for more than 14 years and has shown his work internationally in approximately 140 exhibitions worldwide. The untitled piece pictured below is one of Joshua's stencils. Joshua runs stencil art workshops for a variety of different groups, and over the past four years he has taught over 40 workshops with more than 500 students. These workshops typically last for five to ten weeks, but some are as short as two days depending on the focus or goal of the project. Around 60 to 70% of Joshua's work in this field is with homeless or otherwise disadvantaged youth.

He has held a number of these workshops in locally disadvantaged suburbs where some of the attendees have had multiple offenses for illegal graffiti and are sent for participation by the local council. "Instead of giving them a slap on the wrist or having them go out and cover their own graffiti, they [the council] partner them up with mentors like myself." Joshua is tasked with shaping their perceptions of graffiti and channeling it into more appropriate—and legal— outlets. Other youth often attend Joshua's workshops as part of the school curriculum and will work together to create a mural or another common goal, which may be creating graffiti on an open wall or painting "stobey" (i.e., electrical poles). Adelaide City Council (2013) has given over some areas in the city for both the creation of street art as well as murals. [2]

Joshua has held workshops at a local agency that services people who are experiencing homelessness. These workshops were ongoing and took place over

---

[2] Adelaide City Council. (2013). *Public art.* Retrieved from
http://www.adelaidecitycouncil.com/community/arts-culture/public-art/

the course of 12 weeks at a drop-in center and were open to anyone. The primary focus of this project was to provide a space for people to be creative and an avenue for socialization.

Joshua also ran a seven-week program for the Red Cross with participants' aged 16-25 who had been in and out of prison or juvenile detention. This project incorporated several creative outlets including music production, freestyle graffiti, and stencil art. Students were paired with a mentor in the area that they were most interested in pursuing. For the artists, their work was exhibited in the foyer of the Red Cross, which was later sold at a launch night. The proceeds from this effort directly benefited the participants in that any money received went back into the project and was then evenly allocated across all of the students. The money could then be used to support a particular goal such as the purchase of paint to continue with their art.

Challenges associated with his work are primarily related to issues of involuntary participants and group dynamics. During the process of building rapport and trust, disruptive behavior can emerge. But Joshua states, "Every workshop that I do is different. The demographics are different, and I change my style to match that demographic. If I'm working with students from a private school, I can just come in and give orders because they are quite regimented. But if I'm working with students who have come from harsher environments, you just can't treat them that way because they just won't turn up again. I have to be more of a friend to the students [to gain their trust]." While a refinement of their artwork is one objective of the workshops, participants learn much more. Street art takes time, patience, and dedication and through the workshops and their work with Joshua, participants who are open to the process gain respect for the creation of art and recognize that creating good street art is hard work.

For some participants, these workshops provide the opportunity to gain a skill set—both in art and interpersonally—that can be translated into a way for them to earn an income. Joshua takes this aspect of his work very seriously; he mentors around 30 people—sometimes for years—and has 10 protégées that have all come from the workshops that he runs. He sees the changes that can occur in an individual—from being reunited with estranged parents to the growing self-confidence that comes from working with well-known artists. "I've had kids who have done a full turn around…from putting their tags up everywhere to now working with local councils and actually training other individuals themselves."

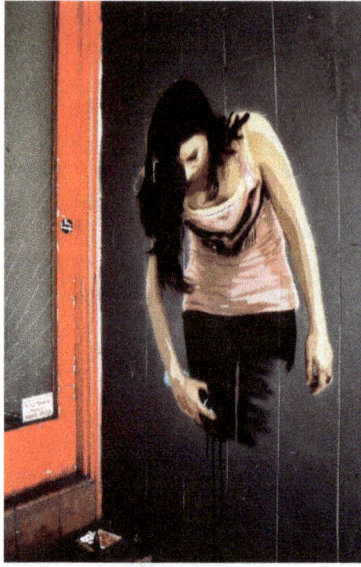

Untitled.
Artist: Joshua Smith.
Location: Adelaide, South Australia.
Photo by: Jill Chonody.

Mural arts

Restorative justice and prison rehabilitation efforts have been incorporated mural arts for some time. One such program, call the *Young New Yorkers*, began as a public art project and is now a court-mandated Brooklyn-based restorative justice program (Barnard, 2013). This project is aimed at 16-17 year old individuals who have been convicted of misdemeanors and offers an alternative to incarceration. Photography, video, illustration, and design were utilized to explore various topics, including the idea of community, choice, responsibility, and leadership (Barnard, 2013). Each of the activities is geared toward creating social connections, and the launch of the program boasts a 100% completion rate for participants (to read more about the first installment, see: http://urbanomnibus.net/2013/07/young-new-yorkers-restorative-justice-through-public-art/). Smaller scale projects that focus on restorative justice can be initiated in the local community that seek to (re-)establish community connections and lead to personal change. For example, a practitioner who works in mandated programs for individuals on probation/parole could incorporate a mural arts project, which could even be painted within the facility.

Similarly, prison based art programs can be found in a number of cities throughout the United States. For example, in Florida, a mural arts program was implemented as a form of art therapy. Based on the therapists' observations, those who participated had better self-esteem and interaction skills as a result of the mural making process (Argue, Bennett, & Gussak, 2009). According to Djurichkovic's (2011) review of prison-based art programs, art is beneficial because the creative process can generate personal empowerment. Given that it is an outlet for emotional expression, mural arts may be particularly useful for those prisoners who suffer from mental illness, an increasingly more common problem.

Additionally, art also provides a positive activity, which in turn benefits administration. These promising results can be one of the ways that mural arts programs can be sold to prison officials who may be hesitant to implement programming due to constrained budgets or philosophical positions regarding criminal justice. Nonetheless, rehabilitative efforts are important for the individual and community alike, and mural arts may be one aspect of those efforts.

Case Example: Facilitating Restorative Justice through Murals

The *Mural Arts Program* in Philadelphia first began in 1984 as part of an anti-graffiti initiative, and led by muralist Jane Golden who quickly recognized the artistic talent of graffiti artists and the transformative power of mural creation. Over the past 30 years, 3,600 murals have been created across the city with a primary focus on community engagement. Current programs include art education, restored spaces and environmental projects, behavioral health initiatives, and restorative justice projects (Mural Arts, 2013).

Robyn Buseman, director of the *Restorative Justice Program*, was interviewed to learn more about it. Reaching over 300 inmates and 200 juveniles each year across a broad context including detention centers, state prison, county jail, and in the community (Family Interrupted, 2013), this program emphasizes "re-entry, reclamation of civic spaces, and the use of art to give voice to people who have consistently felt disconnected from society" (Restorative Justice, 2013, ¶2). The primary goal of the program is to give participants a voice, which can be an empowering experience for individuals who may have never felt like their perspective mattered and who face stigma and discrimination. One program, called *The Guild*, specifically focuses on employment. The program starts in the county jail with art classes and then once released, the men work in the mural arts program and receive additional job training. The goals of this project are twofold: to help ex-offenders find employment in the community and to reduce recidivism. Participants develop relationships with mural arts' staff, artists, and other participants, which can boost their self-confidence. "The guys are really proud to be associated with a respected organization, and when a guy can give back to the community, it is really important."

In addition, the restorative justice component of *Mural Arts* also has projects that occur within the prison system for those who are serving life sentences. This program also works with victim groups and has a close relationship with local agencies. Past and current projects include murals and a community garden. A new mural is planned, which will honor a young man who was murdered, and represents the way in which the program incorporates "stories about how violence impacts the community."

Each year a mural is created that focuses on a social justice issue related to the criminal justice system. The 2013 mural is centered on the theme of mass incarceration, which is aimed at raising public awareness and seeks to humanize people in prison. The 2012 mural, "Family Interrupted," dealt with the impact of incarceration on both families and the community. The creation of the mural was achieved by gathering information from current and ex-inmates, members of the community, adjudicated youth, and those on probation (Family Interrupted, 2013). The effects of incarceration can vary widely—one man who participated in this project just passed his 40th year of incarceration—but many of the youth involved still have the opportunity to spend weekends with their family (Family Interrupted, 2013). Regardless of the amount of time, conviction and incarceration touches everyone. Robyn indicated that the production of a mural is "transformational for them [participants] and her." She gets the opportunity to know her participants and see the many skills that they have to offer and other facets of their personality beyond what has brought them into the system.

References

Mural Arts. (2013). *City of Philadelphia: Mural arts program*. Retrieved from muralarts.org/about.

Family Interrupted. *About*. Retrieved from http://familyinterruptedproject.com/sample-page/.

Restorative Justice. (2013). *City of Philadelphia: Mural arts program*. Retrieved from muralarts.org/programs/restorative-justice.

Behavioral Health

Street Art

The creation of street art in public spaces may provide an ideal outlet for people with mental illness, and this freedom of expression may be particularly beneficial. Free walls could be used to work with individuals and groups—even if the art is only temporary. A group of individuals recovering from mental illness may find release or even catharsis in painting a city wall and expressing their perspective publicly. Taking photographs of both process and product can give the individual a permanent piece of the artwork to take with them from the project. The principles of street art could also be incorporated into an art therapy group either in an inpatient psychiatric unit or as part of an outpatient group. Research suggests that art therapy can improve mood (De Petrillo & Winner, 2005) and that it is an effective approach to practice (Reynolds, Nabors, & Quinlan, 2000). Art therapy is not necessarily superior to other forms of therapy, but it can provide similar results (Reynolds et al., 2000). While the incorporation of street art into art therapy has not be subjected to research, the promising results of art therapy in general suggest that it may be beneficial to participants who are experiencing mental health issues. Using modification, posters, paste-ups, or street art murals within the facility could be used to help participants to explore difficult thoughts, feelings, and experiences. Again, this public expression can be cathartic and help boost self-confidence.

Mural Art

As a way to give back to the community and create an opportunity for self-expression, mural arts projects could also be utilized in psychiatric facilities, hospitals, and clinics. Testa and McCarthy (2004) describe a collaborative mural arts project that took place on an inpatient psychiatric unit with a group of preadolescent boys who had all experienced personal trauma. The focus of the mural was on remembrance of the September 11th attack on the World Trade Center and takes a prominent position in the main hallway of the unit. While the authors did not engage in a formal research process, they report that group solidarity and group identification emerged from the process of collaboration and that their sense of self-efficacy improved. Furthermore, they indicated that "mural making provides a safe and supportive group environment for resolving conflicts and gradually transforming the psychological effects of trauma" (Testa & McCarthy, 2004, p. 40). Mural arts programs can be employed for work with those who have witnessed/experience trauma, individuals experiencing mental illness, and chronic health sufferers. The expressive and collaborative nature of mural arts can be a way to engage with participants or as adjunctive therapy to current practice.

Case Example: Mural Art as an Intervention: Personal Empowerment and Community Connections

The *Porch Light Program* in Philadelphia has a dual focus on community driven art and creating interpersonal connections between participants, artists, and the broader community. Sara Ansell, Program Director of the *Porch Light Program*, was interviewed regarding this program. *Porch Light* has completed 17 large-scale murals with six currently underway. Project goals vary slightly depending on the specific setting for the artwork, but the overarching goal is to create positive change by improving community connectedness. Through increased opportunities for interaction, social barriers in the community can be broken down and a genuine collaboration can occur. Another inherent goal is the advancement of public art in practice given that "it is not typically used in most agencies." Therapists may not think of art as primary intervention, but it can be quite powerful. Sara indicates that a "transformation of their [participants'] perceptions of service, community, and self can occur through the use of art."

The "newness and unexpectedness" of mural arts can catch the "attention and imagination" of participants, which is one of the key benefits to using this approach to practice. This program promotes participants' strengths and through the process of creating the mural, they gain increased confidence to face personal challenges. Additionally, their connection with one another and the broader community is sustained. Some groups continue to meet with one another on a regular basis even after their artwork is complete, and the public mural lives on for all to enjoy.

Sara illustrates how these goals were realized when sharing the following story. Robert[3], who had been notoriously quiet throughout the project, spoke up at the closing ceremony. Robert, who has struggled with substance abuse, explained to the group how he had found his true purpose when he began couching basketball, which he had done for several decades. His successes were numerous, but now, at aged 50 with his coaching days behind him, he indicated that his certificate of participation in *Porch Light* had meant more to him than his past successes because this certificate has made him feel like a valuable member of the community. He knows that the mural will endure, and he felt proud to be part of something larger than himself.

---

[3] Not his real name.

The workshops offered through the *Porch Light Program* vary depending on the goals of the project; however, some communality emerges. First, an artist is embedded in the community, which may be a neighborhood or a specific agency, such as a substance abuse treatment facility, to create cohesiveness and collaboration. Second, workshops typically occur on a weekly basis and include other types of classes for self-expression (e.g., poetry). Third, the creation of the mural is a collaborative process between the artist and participants, which is essential to participant investment and change. Finally, both the mural itself and the workshops are geared toward personal strengths. For example, a current project aimed at educating viewers about autism is working with youth who are living with autism and their families. "This type of artwork seems to be something special to those who are involved. And I'm always amazed by the degree of impact that it can have." To learn more about the Porch Light Program, see: muralarts.org/programs/porch-light.

Benefits and Potential Challenges

One of the primary benefits to using street art in practice with youth is that it has the potential of a ready-made connection. Many young people are in-tune with street artists, such as Banksy or Shephard Fairey, and have an awareness of the underground culture associated with this form of artwork. Whether it is the basis for an educational activity or the framework for an art project, the use of street art can represent a way to engage with adolescents and young adults within their own frame of reference.

Another benefit of street/mural art is the opportunity for personal empowerment and public recognition or appreciation for their artwork. Both temporary and permanent art pieces may serve as a source of pride and enhance self-esteem. Similarly, the use of public art can improve the community and its members' sense of pride and ownership. Well-placed murals that are created through the participation of residents can further those connections.

A potential challenge to mural arts is garnering support within the community and attaining permission to create large-scale murals. The desires of the community should take precedence over the goals of practitioners. Residents may view the practitioner as an outsider who does not have the best interest of the community at heart. Establishing trust and collaborative relationships will be essential to the success of a community mural art project.

Ethical Considerations

The primary ethical issue when considering street art is the legality of the efforts. Obviously, engaging vulnerable individuals in unlawful behavior is not advisable. As more cities around the globe are embracing the aesthetic contributions of street art, legal walls may become more common. If that is not the case in one's local area, there are creative ways that this challenge might be skirted. For example, seeking out a local business that may be willing to allow the creation of spray paint art may offer an alternative approach. Or perhaps participants still in school could be organized to raise awareness about a particular topic, and then, with the help of the principal, use posters in the hallways to illustrate the issue. In other words, the basic principles of street art can be the framework for developing activities that are consistent with legal parameters, but still achieve project goals of personal empowerment, artistic expression, and raising awareness.

Another ethical issue that should be considered is credit for contributions to the artwork. When large-scale pieces are generated with a significant number of people involved in various ways (e.g., input on design, drawing, painting, etc), acknowledgment of their role should be included in some way. This inclusion can mean a great deal to the contributors who may now feel like a real "artist." When the final product is drawn and painted, a delicate balance on how best to make those acknowledgements will need to be negotiated. Regardless of how this is ultimately resolved, the discussion should occur up front with all those involved, including local agencies, funders or organizers of the mural, and all of the artists and participants.

Tips for Practitioners

1. **Use photographs to illustrate the process of making public artwork.** These photographs can then be used to create a memory book of the project that participants can take away as a keepsake of their participation. These albums can also include drawings, writings, and mementos, which may represent personal or group progression throughout the project (Testa & McCarthy, 2004).

2. **Create collaborative engagements with local street artists who are interested in creating legal, public artwork and engaging with the community.** The innovative approach taken in Australia to work with youth, particularly those who had interaction with law enforcement, to create public works of art shows promise. Skill development, artistic expression, and visibility in the public may be just a few of the benefits that could emerge from a street art engagement project.

3. **Carefully consider competing interests of creating a professional artistic image and a fully participant-driven creation.** Various stakeholders may have sway in how this process is propelled and thus how the final piece looks. However, the higher the degree of participation and decision making that can be given to participants, the more likely they are to gain from the experience in terms of personal empowerment. An alternate approach to creating one large mural may be the use of tiles painted by many participants, which are then used to form a large mosaic type mural.

4. **Utilize available guides to help with public art implementation.** While many resources are available for purchase, many informative and practical resources are accessible for free on the Internet. See the *Readings and Resources* section for some of these.

5. **An alternative to creating public art is viewing it with others.** Graffiti is ubiquitous for those dwelling in urban areas and not an uncommon experience across suburban or rural landscapes. "It provides the opportunity to discuss the social roles that art can play and the legal issues it can raise about the rights and responsibilities of the artist" (Whitehead, 2004, p. 26). Whether it is graffiti or other forms of public

art, this approach may be used to engage participants in a critical discussion of history, community strengths and issues, art, or culture. Given the widespread use of smart phones, participants could capture photographs of public artwork, either as an organized group effort or a solo project, to be deconstructed later. These discussions may then be used to develop community projects or other explorations that may help participants develop group cohesion, collaboration, or personal empowerment.

6. **When creating a mural with a group of participants, consider how funding can be utilized as part of the long-term maintenance of the art and how participants may be engaged in that process.** Given exposure to elements and possibility of vandalism, efforts should be made to keep the mural in good condition. Fund raising within the community may offer one way to achieve this goal. If members of that particular area enjoy the artwork, then they may be willing to make a small contribution to help with its ongoing maintenance. An event that features both the mural and the artists who created it may be one way to generate both funding and support for the project.

7. **Street art and community murals can be shared with key stakeholders by creating blogs, self-published books (e.g., *Blurb*), or hosting an e-book on agency websites.** If the goal of the project is to reach the wider community, including those who are in a position of power, then the incorporation of technology may facilitate that purpose. For example, if working with a group of individuals who are experiencing mental illness with the aim of providing education and decreasing social stigma, then one might seek to include images of the mural making process on a blog. The link to this blog could then be sent out to local agencies, political figures, and posted on social media sites. Free blogs are available through *Blogger* and support both images and text.

8. **While this chapter has primarily focused on painting walls, other forms of public art could offer similar benefits for participants.** This may include the creation of mosaics, sculpture, or performance pieces. Moreover, found objects could be used to create a mural or alternative public spaces could be painted, such as benches or telephone poles.

9. **Involving the local community is essential when considering a mural arts project.** Gude and Pounds (2013) offer a number of excellent tips on how this process can be achieved, including: creating a dialogue, documenting community involvement, experiencing the site, building trust, and setting goals (for the full list, see: www.cpag.net/guide/1/1_pages/1_2.htm).

10. **Additional research on how public art can lead to change is needed.** When undertaking a new project, consider collecting data to document change or collaborating with faculty at a local university to help with the research process. Outcome based research for these approaches are largely missing, and studying the way that these endeavors facilitate change can lead to improvement or refinement. Chapter 14, *Approaches to Evaluation: How to Measure Change when Utilizing Creative*

Approaches, provides a starting point for thinking about how evaluation can be included in a new project.

Recommended Readings and Resources

Banksy. (2006). *Bansky: Wall and piece.* London: Random House.

Borrup, T. (2011). *The creative community builder's handbook: How to transform communities using local assets, art, and culture.* New York: Fieldstone Alliance.

Chicago Public Art Group. (2013). *Community public art guide: Making murals, mosaics, sculptures, and spaces.* Available at: http://www.cpag.net/guide/.

Golden, J., Rice, R., & Kinney, M. Y. (2002). *Philadelphia murals and the stories they tell.* Philadelphia, PA: Temple University Press.

Gude, O., & Pounds, J. (2013). *Community engagement: Chicago public art group's steps for creating community designed places.* Available at: www.cpag.net/guide/1/1_pages/1_2.htm.

Humboldt Park Mural Arts Program Enrichment Project. (2013). *Teaching toolkit.* Available at: http://architreasures.org/wp-content/uploads/2013/04/HPMAP-Curriculum_Reduced.pdf.

Lazarides, S. (2008). *Outsiders: Art by people.* London: Century.

Russell, R. (2004). A beginner's guide to public art. *Art Education, 57*(4), 19-24.

Tápies, X. A. (2007). *Street art and the war on terror: How the world's best graffiti artists said no to the Iraq war.* E. Mathieson (Ed.). London: Rebellion Books.

The Heidelberg Project. (2013). *Changing lives through art since 1986.* Available at: http://www.heidelberg.org/.

Zander, M. J. (2004). Instructional resources: Murals as documents of social history. *Art Education, 57*(5), 25-31.

References

Argue, J., Bennett, J., & Gussak, D. (2009). Transformation through negotiation: Initiating the inmate mural arts program. *The Arts in Psychotherapy, 36*(5), 313-319.

Austin, J. (2010). More to see than a canvas in a white cube: For an art in the streets. *City: Analysis of Urban Trends, Culture, Theory, Policy, and Action, 14*(1-2), 33-47.

Barnard, R. (2013). Young New Yorkers: Restorative justice through public art. *The Architectural League's urban omnibus: The culture of citymaking.* Retrieved from http://urbanomnibus.net/2013/07/young-new-yorkers-restorative-justice-through-public-art/.

Buffington, M. L. (2007). Art to bring about change: The work of Tyree Guyton. *Art Education, 60,* 25-32.

De Petrillo, L., & Winner, E. (2005). Does art improve mood? A test of a key assumption underlying art therapy. *Art Therapy: Journal of the Art Therapy Association, 22*(4), 205-212.

Djurichkovic, A. (2011). "Art in prisons:" A literature review of the philosophies and impacts of visual arts programs for correctional populations. *Arts access Australia*. University of Technology Sydney. Retrieved from http://epress.lib.uts.edu.au/research/bitstream/handle/2100/1212/ArtinPrisons_Djurichkovic.pdf?sequence=3.

Fradella, L. (2005). Murals as storytellers. *School Arts: The Art Education Magazine for Teachers, 104*, 25-27.

Gastman, R., Neelon, C., & Smyrski, A. (2007). *Street world: Urban art and culture from five continents.* London: Thames & Hudson.

Howze, R. (2008). *Stencil nation: Graffiti, community, and art.* San Francisco, CA: Manic D Press.

Hutzel, K. (2007). Reconstructing a community, reclaiming a playground: A participatory action research study. *Studies in Art Education: A Journal of Issues and Research, 48*(3), 299-315.

Iveson, K. (2013). Cities within the city: Do-it-yourself urbanism and the right to the city. *International Journal of Urban and Regional Research, 37*(3), 941-956.

Kramer, R. (2010). Painting with permission: Legal graffiti in New York City. *Ethnography, 11*, 235-253.

Marschall, S. (1999). A critical investigation into the impact of community mural art. *Transformation, 40*, 55-86.

Marschall, S. (2002). Sites of identity and resistance: Urban community murals and rural wall decoration in South Africa. *African Arts, 35*, 40-53.

McGrogan, M. (2008). Art on the street. *History Today, 58*, 34-36.

Moss, K. L. (2010). Cultural representation in Philadelphia murals: Images of resistance and sites of identity negotiation. *Western Journal of Communication, 74*(4), 372-395.

MTA. (2013). Arts for transit and urban design. Retrieved from www.mta.info/mta/aft/about/.

Reynolds, M. W., Nabors, L., & Quinlan, A. (2000). The effectiveness of art therapy: Does it work? *Art Therapy: Journal of the American Art Therapy Association, 17*(3), 207-213.

Testa, N., & McCarthy, J. B. (2004). The use of murals in preadolescent inpatient groups: An art therapy approach to cumulative trauma. *Art Therapy: Journal of the American Art Therapy Association, 21*(1), 38-41.

Whitehead, J. L. (2004). Graffiti: The use of the familiar. *Art Education, 57*(6), 25-32.

Chapter 4: Singing: Creating Harmony in Mind and Body

Barbra Teater

Introduction

The Oxford Dictionary (2013) defines song as "a short poem or other sets of words set to music or meant to be sung," and singing as to "make musical sounds with the voice, especially words with a set tune." Singing is one form of music where words are expressed through a vocal sound. Singing and the use of song are parts of human nature that are open to everyone and valued in all cultures. Singing has been found to not only elicit emotional responses within the singer, but to contribute to the singer's physical, emotional, and social health and well-being (Clift, Hancox, Staricoff, & Whitmore, 2008). The physical, emotional, and social benefits of singing have consistently been found across different populations, such as homeless individuals (Bailey & Davidson, 2002), middle-class individuals (Bailey & Davidson, 2005), individual and choral singers (Beck, Gottfried, Hall, Cisler, & Bozeman, 2006; Grape, Sandgren, Hansson, Ericson, & Theorell, 2003; Kreutz et al., 2004), female prisoners (Silber, 2005), people with enduring mental health difficulties (Clift, 2010), individuals with chronic respiratory disease (Lord et al., 2010), and older adults (Cohen et al., 2006, 2007; Teater & Baldwin, 2012).

This chapter explores the use of singing as a therapeutic source to enhance physical and emotional well-being with a focus on the use of group singing versus individual singing given the greater social benefits associated with the it. Beginning with an overview of music, singing, and song and how they are important to human nature and expression across cultures provides a framework for a discussion around singing as a therapeutic source. Exploring the benefits of singing, as evidenced through research with various populations, and a few examples of how it is implemented in practice illustrates the usefulness of this approach. Challenges to using singing in practice are explored as well as ethical considerations, and tips for practitioners are provided. The chapter concludes with a description of a community singing group for older adults.

Music, Singing, and the Use of Song

Singing and song have served as a form of human expression for centuries. Music, in particular, but often singing and song, are present within many facets of our daily lives from music heard on the radio, on television, at parties and gatherings, in office buildings, and while being on hold on the telephone. Music, singing, and song play an even larger part in defining different cultures in terms of their use in ceremonial and celebratory occasions, battle songs, religious hymns, chants, marching songs, and national anthems (Unwin, Kenny, & Davis, 2002). Music, singing, and song can also be defined or labeled based on its creation and emergence through different geographical areas or cultural groups, such as Bluegrass, Country, Hip Hop, Salsa, Calypso, or Gaelic, just to name a few. In this sense, music, singing, and song can be directly related to one's identity. For example, Ruud (1998) argues:

> [M]usic plays an important role in the construction of identity within the mediascape that surrounds us from birth to death. Music can serve as raw material for building values and life orientations, as a way to anchor important relationships to other people, as a way of framing our situatedness in a certain time and space, and as a way to position ourselves within our cultures and thus make explicit out ethnicity, gender, and class. It also provides important 'peak' or transcendental experiences that may strengthen the formation of identity in the sense that we feel meaning, purpose, and significance in our life (p. 47-48).

Listening to music of one's culture has repeatedly been found to elicit emotional responses in individuals across cultural groups (Bigand, Vieillard, Madurell, Marozeau, & Dacquet, 2005; Juslin & Laukka, 2003). The act of listening to music has also been found to activate brain regions that stimulate reward and motivation (Blood & Zatorre, 2001). The influence of music, in particular the lyrics of a song, has been found to serve as a coping mechanism for individuals when experiencing difficult situations (Ahmadi, 2011). Yet, there is a difference between listening to music and participating in the making of music through singing. Although both listening and singing have been found to enhance the mood of the individual (Chlan, 1995; McKinney et al., 1997), the effects have been more robust for the singer over the listener (Unwin et al., 2002).

The use of music in therapeutic settings has existed for centuries such as attempting to drive out evil forces to overcome illness (Bailey & Davidson, 2003a), but the use of music therapy in the United States as a formal method and academic discipline emerged in the 1950s (Ruud, 1997). Music therapy can comprise the use of singing, listening to, or discussing music to reach a goal, such as to enhance mental functioning, quality of life, or even the motor skills of the individual. Singing, as one form of music therapy, may be in a one-on-one setting or a group setting through a choir or community singing group. The implementation of individual or group singing as a therapeutic source may be delivered by a trained music therapist or aspects of "music therapy" can be integrated into other forms of therapeutic practices, such as social work, counseling, community work, and mental health nursing.

This chapter is focused on the use of group singing, particularly with adults, as a therapeutic source due to the growing evidence of the benefits in terms of enhancing physical, emotional, and social health and well-being, which is discussed in more detail in the next section. Whereas singing and listening to music has been found to enhance mood and elicit emotional responses, the benefits of group singing extend beyond the individual emotional benefits into group and communal benefits. According to Vink (2001), music therapists have argued that:

> [M]usic cannot be considered as medicine as it is not merely the music from which the client benefits. Other factors contribute to the therapeutic effect as well, such as the group interaction, the interaction with the music and the therapeutic alliance (p. 145).

This argument acknowledges that implementing group singing as a source of therapy not only requires a focus on the music, but also the group effects and the role of the facilitator, leader, or conductor.

Singing as a Source of Therapy

Several theories have emerged to explain why singing, including singing in groups, yields physical, emotional, and social benefits to the singer (Clift et al., 2008). Csikszentmihalyi's (2002) theory of "flow" is focused on the process whereby individuals are entrenched in an activity to the point that they are lost in their work. The individual is fully concentrated on the task at hand to the point that there is no concentration left to focus on other things. This theory was applied to singing by Bailey and Davidson (2003b) who recognized that singing requires both concentration and skill; thus, it can enable someone to reach a state of flow by losing themselves in singing. This process removes negative emotions and feelings, such as depression and anxiety, or other preoccupations.

Other theorists and researchers (Cohen et al., 2006; Flood, 2006) have argued that engaging in creative activities, such as group singing, can enhance health and well-being among older adults by giving them a sense of control and opportunities for social engagement. In this sense, it is not necessarily the act of singing that creates the benefits, but the act of participating in a creative activity, particularly with others, that contributes to one's sense of self and their relationship with others.

The Benefits of Singing

The research evidence for the benefits of singing is continually expanding and includes studies that look at individual and group singing, auditioned and amateur singing groups, and newly created and long-standing groups. Clift et al. (2008) conducted a systematic mapping and review of the research on the relationship between singing and health. They included exploratory studies, which comprised qualitative approaches or subjective information gathered from the singers, and hypothesis-testing studies, which encompassed standardized measurements and scales and/or the collection of objective measures of biological or physiological functioning. In regard to the exploratory studies, the benefits to physical, emotional, and social health and well-being were found to include the following perceived benefits (Clift et al., 2008):

- Physical relaxation and release of physical tension;
- Emotional release and reduction of feelings of stress;
- A sense of happiness, positive mood, joy, elation and feeling high;
- A sense of greater personal, emotional and physical wellbeing;
- An increased sense of arousal and energy;
- Stimulation of cognitive capacities–attention, concentration, memory, learning;
- A sense of being absorbed in an activity which draws on multiple capacities of the body and the mind;
- A sense of collective bonding through coordinated activity following the same pulse;
- The potential for personal contact with others who are like-minded and the development of personal supportive friendships and constructive collaborative relationships;
- A sense of contributing to a product which is greater than the sum of its parts;
- A sense of personal transcendence beyond mundane and everyday realities, being put in touch with a sense of beauty and something beyond words, which is moving or good for the soul;
- An increased sense of self-confidence and self-esteem;
- A sense of therapeutic benefit in relation to long-standing psychological and social problems (e.g., depression, a history of abuse, problems with drugs and alcohol, social disadvantage);
- A sense of contributing to the wider community through public performance;
- A sense of exercising systems of the body through the physical exertion involved in singing – especially the lungs;
- A sense of disciplining the skeletal-muscular system through the adoption of good posture; and
- Being engaged in a valued, meaningful, worthwhile activity that gives a sense of purpose and motivation (p. 5-6).

Several researchers have attempted to conceptualize the perceived benefits of singing into a model of distinct factors. For example, Hills and Argyle (1998) found the perceived benefits of singing fall into five groups: well-being, mystical experience, social benefits, entertainment, and intellectual/musical benefits. Clift and Hancox (2001) found perceived benefits of group singing to fall within six groups: well-being and relaxation; breathing and posture; social benefits; spiritual benefits; emotional benefits; and heart and immune system benefits. Finally, Bailey and Davidson (2002, 2005) have developed a model that incorporates the benefits of group singing, which includes four groups: clinical-type benefits; social benefits; benefits associated with public performance; and cognitive stimulation.

The benefits of singing have also been explored through more objective studies that use biological measurements, standardized measures, or use a comparison group. Studies using standardized measures of health and well-being, such as the General Health Questionnaire (GHQ), have continually found positive results among older adults in terms of physical and mental health (Cohen et al., 2006, 2007). Other studies have used standardized measures, such as the Profile of Mood States questionnaire (POMS), to explore the extent to which singing affects mood and stress. A randomized control trial with 28 adults found that 13 weeks of music therapy resulted in a decrease in mood disturbance as measured by the POMS (McKinney et al., 1997). Enhanced mood was also found among 20 mechanically ventilated patients when exposed to music listening (Chlan, 1995). Although this chapter focuses on the act of singing versus listening to music, the research has found that both singing and listening result in enhanced mood, but the results for those individuals within singing groups, results indicate a greater effect (Unwin et al., 2002).

Biological measurements, such as cortisol levels or salivary immunoglobulin A (slgA), have been used to determine the potential health benefits of singing. Cortisol is a steroid hormone released in response to stress, and slgA is an antibody that fights against infection. The results of changes in cortisol levels have varied based on the research study. For example, Beck, Cesario, Yousefi, and Enamoto (2000) took cortisol levels of choral singers before and after rehearsals and performance and found cortisol levels to reduce after rehearsals, but to increase after performance; however, Kreutz et al. (2004) found no change in cortisol levels before and after a choral rehearsal (Clift et al., 2008). The studies that have used slgA have found that an increase in slgA in saliva occurs post singing (Beck et al., 2000; Beck et al., 2006; Kuhn, 2002; Kreutz, et al., 2004). Although these findings are positive in terms of health benefits for singers, there is no evidence that this is sustained in the long term.

The Use of Singing in Practice

The way in which singing is incorporated into practice will depend on the aim(s) and goal(s) that the practitioner (and individual/group) intends to achieve. For example, a goal of increasing social contact for socially excluded and isolated older adults might result in a one-hour singing session at a local community center where the participants sing along to a pre-recorded music and use a singing book that lists the words. If the goal is to enhance physical health, then individuals might be tasked with a choreographed song. If the goal is to enhance breathing and lung capacity, then the sessions might include warm up sessions where individuals exercise their lungs through specific singing exercises. Additionally, the use of singing might be the main intervention piece, for example to enhance breathing and lung capacity. Alternatively, it might be the catalyst to reach other goals, such as enhancing social connections and interactions. Several examples of how singing has been used in practice are reviewed here.

Bailey and Davidson (2003a) describe an amateur singing group called *The Homeless Choir*, which was developed by a soup kitchen volunteer who had no specialist training in music nor in music therapy. The volunteer was a member of a choir and believed that the benefits and rewards that he had gained as a choir member may be beneficial for homeless men as well. The volunteer invited the men to join a newly formed choir, and he specified that there was no prior training or knowledge of group singing required. The choir started with three men, but quickly grew to twenty. Since the choir was developed, they have performed over 1,000 concerts, with the first being in a subway terminal, have recorded several CDs, and have appeared on television. Bailey and Davidson (2003a) have found that the quality of life of the men have been greatly enhanced through their participation in the choir. At the time of their evaluation, choir members were in stable housing and many had paid employment.

Whereas *The Homeless Choir* is an ongoing choir with no set time limit, other singing interventions are time-limited. Davidson and Fedele (2011) describe a six-week singing group for older adults with dementia (aged 70 and over) residing in a residential care unit and their professional caregivers, and other older adults with dementia who live in the community and their informal carers. Community music educators and therapists developed the program, and one facilitator with extensive experience in leading singing groups delivered the sessions. The facilitator chose the songs for each session with some input from participants, including Hebrew and Yiddish songs since many participants were Jewish. The groups met for two hours each week for six weeks. Davidson and Fedele's (2011) evaluation of the program yielded positive outcomes for the people with dementia as reported by the caregivers, the facilitator, and the researchers, including lucidity, improved interaction during the session, and carry-over memory from one week to the next.

The above program is based on the work of Bailey and Davidson (2005) and Davidson and Faulkner (2010) who have devised a systematic approach to working with groups of older adults and people with disabilities. Their work has suggested the following approaches for facilitators/practitioners to consider when using singing in group settings (as cited in Davidson and Fedele, 2011):

1. Begin by warming the voice and body with gentle vocalization and physical exercises;
2. As the session progresses, encourage more vigorous breathing/diaphragmatic support work and physical stretching;
3. Connect participants with musical games for technical and social impact – tongue-twisters, rounds, rhythmic movement;
4. Make sure that all of the above are undertaken at the singer's personal level of comfort – chairs should always be available should anyone feel tired, dizzy, or uncomfortable;
5. Select a range of invigorating as well as soothing and comforting repertoire;
6. Provide both familiar and new repertoire;
7. Encourage creative participation in song – writing and harmonization, with unaccompanied and accompanied songs;
8. Encouraging critical reflective listening, with attention to pitch-matching, good one quality, and support of the singing tone, using legato, staccato, and florid exercises;
9. Always move at a comfortable pace, with opportunities for hydration, rest, and refreshment breaks to encourage recovery and social exchange;

10. Introduce a program of performance opportunities, which encourages memorization and motivation towards ongoing singing out into the community;

11. Use strong singing facilitators who have a sound knowledge of physical and psychological concerns of the cohort to lead the groups; and

12. Encourage the leader's use of humor and fun to stimulate participants (p. 404).

Although the suggestions above have been used with singing groups for older adults and people with disabilities, each practitioner will need to match the specifics of the sessions with the aims and goals of the singing group as well as the specific characteristics and needs of the group.

Benefits and Potential Challenges

As stated above, research evidence indicates clear benefits to the use of singing when aimed at enhancing physical, emotional, and social well-being among individuals and groups and extends across a variety of settings and different individual and group characteristics and traits. In addition to the benefits of using singing in terms of outcomes for participants, there are also benefits to choosing this type of method to incorporate into practice. This section discusses both the benefits and challenges to incorporating singing in practice.

Singing is an activity that can be used with individuals of all ages, across cultural groups, with varying levels of singing ability, and in many different settings. As discussed at the beginning of this chapter, music, singing, and song are present in everyday life, and many individuals will have knowledge of singing and will have preferred songs and types of music. Therefore, the use of singing could be applicable in nearly every therapeutic setting.

As singing and song are common across cultures, access to this method can be quite simple. Individuals may be able to bring songs to the sessions or the practitioner may select songs based on the individual or group. Singing also does not require accompanying music or song lyrics as many individuals know songs from memory or can create and write songs themselves. Additionally, singing can occur across different settings, from an office setting, to one's home, to the outdoors, to a rehearsal studio, or to a performance hall. Although many individuals may have had training in singing through school, church, or community choirs, those individuals without training are still capable of and familiar with singing; thus, it needs little to no introduction or training on what it entails. Therefore, in addition to being an easily accessible method, the use of singing may also require few resources.

Another benefit to the use of singing is that the practitioner may have set a particular aim as the result of singing, such as enhanced self-esteem, yet the outcomes will likely expand beyond that goal to include other benefits. For example, a study by Teater and Baldwin (2012) found that not only did participants in a community-based singing group report feeling physically and emotionally healthier by participating in the program, but they also reported that they made friends and their social connections and interactions enhanced greatly to the point that they were participating in social activities with other members outside of the one-hour singing session. Two participants also reported stopping prescription medication for depression and discontinuing alcohol use. Therefore, the use of singing may support the practitioner in achieving particular aims and goals, but the practitioner may want to look out for unintended benefits as well.

The main challenge to incorporating singing is that it is not for everyone. Some individuals do not enjoy singing, do not want to sing, or are embarrassed or shy when singing around others. This could be that someone merely does not like to sing or that s/he fears being judged by others around her/him or has negative perceptions of her/his own voice (Chong, 2010). When faced with this challenge, the practitioner may need to educate the individual on the varying abilities of people to sing, the benefits of singing, and how to manage the possibility of being judged by others if in a group setting. If the individual continues to decline the offer of singing, then the practitioner should respect her/his right to self-determination and select an alternative method.

Another challenge is understanding and acknowledging group dynamics when using group singing. Just as with any formed group, practitioners can expect groups of singers to experience the five stages of Tuckman's (1965) group development: forming; storming; norming; performing; and adjourning. This involves acknowledging that groups experience a "honeymoon" or *forming* stage at the beginning when they are getting to know one another, yet enter a *storming* stage when they become comfortable with each other and begin to challenge one another and establish roles within the group. The group moves into the *norming* stage once they have established boundaries, roles, and norms, which then feeds into the *performing* stage where they are most productive in terms of reaching their goal. Finally, *adjourning* is when the group ends and there is a need for reflection on what was learnt and achieved as well as an acknowledgment of the end and loss of the group.

Finally, just as singing can be a benefit in terms of limited resources required for its use, on the opposite end of the spectrum, some situations might require a vast amount of resources. This is particularly the case for group singing where the practitioner will need to access a venue that can support the singing (rehearsals and performance), and consider the cost of a facilitator or conductor, printed and copyrighted materials, marketing, refreshments, transportation, and any accompanying artists. The practitioner may decide that s/he will need to charge for membership to the group or the practitioner may seek external funding to support the group. This will most likely depend on the aims and goals of the singing group and the characteristics of the group.

Ethical Considerations

The use of singing, particularly group singing, tends to be with vulnerable or at-risk individuals or with a group of individuals who share a common interest or need, for example a singing group for homeless men, a community singing group for socially isolated older adults, or a performing choir of people with enduring mental health problems. Given that the individuals may be vulnerable, harm reduction should be considered. This can be accomplished in part by establishing clear rules and guidelines for group members, the practitioner, and voluntary workers. Rules around confidentiality should be made explicit as well as examples regarding the limits of confidentiality. There should be rules around mutual respect for one another and exploration of appropriate and inappropriate behavior and expectations.

As singing may be expressed differently between participants, it is important to acknowledge differences and respect the ways in which singers may express themselves (where appropriate). Group dynamics may play an important role if one or a few members of the group take charge and overshadow quiet or timid members. It is important for the practitioner to keep a balance within the group where members are able to express themselves, but individual expression is not interfering in the achievement of the group's goal. The practitioner will need to consider the balance between mutual and individual benefit.

Another ethical consideration is in terms of any materials (performances, concerts, recorded songs) produced by the individual or group. Individuals should be informed from the beginning as to whether there are any charges to participate and, if so, how their money will be spent. If there are entry charges to performances and concerts, the members should know how any profit will be used. Group members should agree to recordings of rehearsals, performances, and concerts ahead of time, and any member who does not wish to be recorded should have the right to decline participation in that event.

Finally, the goal(s) for the use of singing with the individual or group should be made explicit from the beginning and should be kept at the forefront of all work and activities. The practitioner should continually evaluate the extent to which the work is moving the individual or group toward that goal and revise the work as necessary.

Tips for Practitioners

1. **Why use singing? What is your main goal?** Before implementing singing, you should first establish the aim(s) and goal(s). Are you incorporating singing in order to enhance self-esteem? Alleviate depression? Enhance social contact? Increase lung capacity? The list of perceived benefits, as found through the systematic mapping of the research by Clift et al. (2008), could be a good starting point in determining the main aims of using singing. Once those are established, then you are better prepared to design the intervention and you have a clear rationale for its use.

2. **Will you use individual singing or group singing? Will the individual(s) need to audition?** Your established goals should indicate whether you are going to use singing on an individual basis or if singing will be implemented with a group of people. For example, if your aim were to increase social contact, then you would naturally use group over individual singing. You will also need to establish if the singers will audition or if it is open to everyone. If your aim is to form a choir that will preform to paid audiences and the songs the choir sings requires harmonies and solos then you may be more inclined to audition the group members. You will also need to determine who auditions the members and the criteria for inclusion and exclusion.

3. **If you are using group singing, what is the minimum and maximum number of individuals? What are the characteristics or traits of the individuals that enable them to have commonality?** When creating singing groups, you will need to establish the size of the group. This might be based on resources, such as space, or might be directly related to your goals, such as numbers of singers in a four-part choir. You will also need to determine any specific characteristics or traits of the group members, such as age, gender, ethnicity, geographical location, or specific need. Once the specific characteristics and traits of the group have been established, you will need to consider whether the group is open or closed to "outsiders" or people who do not meet the criteria.

4. **What songs will you use? Who will select them? How will they be used? Will they use dance or other movements?** You will need to determine the type of song to use with the group. Will the facilitator/conductor/practitioner choose the songs or will the individual or group be able to select songs? How will the music be played to the individual or group? Will you need an accompanist? Will the songs be choreographed or require any movement?

5. **Will you have a facilitator? Conductor? Will this person be trained or untrained? Paid or unpaid? Should the facilitator hold specific characteristics or traits?** You will need to determine if there will be one person assigned to lead the group or if this role is shared. Will the facilitator/conductor/practitioner be trained or can this person be untrained? If trained, what type of training will be required? Will the person be paid or will the work be on a voluntary basis? If the singers are to hold specific characteristics or traits, should you also require this of the facilitator/conductor/practitioner? For example, if you are holding a community singing group with participants from a particular racial/ethnic group, should the facilitator also have a similar background?

6. **How will you build rapport among the group members?** If you are holding a singing group, you will need to consider group dynamics and how you attempt to create rapport and a sense of solidarity among the group members. What will be the facilitator/conductor/practitioner's role in creating a sense of community among the group and how will the facilitator participate in this process?

7. **Where will the singing take place? How long will the singing last? Are the singing sessions time-limited or open-ended? To what extent is the session structured?** You will need to determine the location of the singing and a time frame for each session. Is the group time limited, for example, six weekly sessions only, or is the group open-ended with no set end date? You will also need to consider the extent to which each session is structured. Is there a set agenda for each session or can it vary from session to session?

8. **What are the resource implications?** What resources do you need to use singing as a method and to achieve your goals? You will need to consider physical, material, and human resources as well as the financial implications for each, such as meeting space, printed copies of music,

equipment to play music, cost of copyrighted material, cost of a facilitator, and cost of transportation and refreshments.

9. **How will you address issues of safety?** This is particularly important when working with groups as you will need to consider how to ensure the safety of all participants. It will be important to look at health and safety policies within your work place as well as the setting where the singing occurs. You should have policies in regard to confidentiality and risk, and these should be made known to the members at the beginning of the work together.

10. **Have you matched the singing activities to the needs, wants, and abilities of your group?** When working with groups, you will need to consider the extent to which your selection of music and songs and the structure of each session meet the needs, wants, and abilities of the group members. Again, you will refer to your aims and consider the characteristics and traits of the group members. Are the singing activities interesting to group members? Are the members physically and emotionally able to participate? Do the members get a sense of perceived benefits through participation? You can evaluate the extent to which these factors are being met through formal and informal evaluations and reviews of the activities.

A Case Example: Community Singing Group for Older Adults

Golden Oldies (www.golden-oldies.org.uk) is a charitable organization in the United Kingdom that provides community-based singing sessions to older adults who are socially isolated as well as individuals with learning difficulties and people with dementia. The *Golden Oldies* program is based on the idea that singing is good for you and that there are physical, emotional, and social benefits to group singing. *Golden Oldies* have three main aims: to reduce social isolation and increase social contact; to provide an environment for participants to make new friends; and to encourage participants to have activities and things to look forward to (Teater & Baldwin, 2012).

The structure of *Golden Oldies* is quite simple as the program provides an environment and resources for older adults to get together and sing songs from the 50s, 60s, and 70s for one hour a week. The sessions are led by a paid facilitator who brings official *Golden Oldies* songbooks to each session for the "Goldies" to use as well as a CD player to play the pre-recorded music. The charity has worked with local governments and voluntary agencies to receive funding to transport older adults to the sessions as well as to have the use of community-based facilities. For example, many weekly sessions are held in a community hall that is located within a sheltered housing estate. Many of the residents are able to walk to the community center whereas others have difficulties in mobility and require assistance from a friend or the estate's warden. Other individuals are transported in from neighboring areas and the charity provides the funding for the transportation cost.

Once at the location, participants gather in a single room where they mingle. Refreshments of tea, coffee, and cakes are often available, and volunteers take charge of setting up, serving, and clearing afterwards. The session leader begins the session with a pre-selected song and will then ask for requests throughout the hour. Many participants will stand and sing, move, sway, or dance and interlock their arms or hands with their friends. Other participants may stay seated. There are also those occasions when someone connects to the song being played and becomes tearful, closes their eyes, or plays out their thoughts, which were stimulated by the song. For example, I have seen a woman fold up her sweater, hold it in her arms and rock it like a baby, and I have also seen a woman who has difficulty walking, stand up, brace herself against a table and move her feet to dance to the music. As the *Golden Oldies* is a community-based singing group and not a choir, there is great variation in the singing; there are those that sing in tune and those that belt out the words off-key. It does not matter as they are all singing together!

The *Golden Oldies* participants are mainly comprised of white women, but the charity has since expanded to recruit more men and people from Black and Minority Ethnic (BME) backgrounds. The newly formed BME group in the southwest of England was carefully considered in terms of the choice of music that would be played at each session and the person who would facilitate the sessions. The charity was able to appoint a BME female who was very familiar with the local community.

An evaluation of the *Golden Oldies* program by Teater and Baldwin (2012) found that between 73.1 and 98.3% of participants ($N = 120$) agreed or strongly agreed that the *Golden Oldies* contributed to their self-development, health, and sense of community as well as revealing a statistically significant increase in self-reported health prior to participation in the program to the time of the study. Qualitative data revealed that the singing group helped to reduce social isolation and increase social contact where the participants were making friends through the singing group and becoming more socially active outside of the *Golden Oldies* sessions.

Recommended Readings and Resources

Chong, H. J. (2010). Do we all enjoy singing? A content analysis of non-vocalists' attitudes towards singing. *The Arts in Psychotherapy, 37*(2), 120-124.

Clift, S., & Hancox, G. (2010). The significance of choral singing for sustaining psychosocial wellbeing: Findings from a survey of choristers in England, Australia and Germany. *Music Performance Research, 3*(1), 79-96.

Clift, S., Hancox, G., Staricoff, R., & Whitmore, C. (2008). *Singing and health: Summary of a systematic mapping and review of non-clinical research.* Sidney De Haan Research Centre for Arts and Health: Cantebury Christ Church University.

Horn, S. (2013). *Imperfect harmony: Finding happiness singing with others.* Chapel Hill, NC: Algonquin Books of Chapel Hill.

Teater, B., & Baldwin, M. (2012). Singing for successful ageing: The perceived benefits of participating in the Golden Oldies community-arts programme. *British Journal of Social Work*. Published online first at http://bjsw.oxfordjournals.org/content/early/2012/07/02/bjsw.bcs095. doi: 10.1093/bjsw/bcs095.

References

Ahmadi, F. (2011). Song lyrics and the alternation of self-image. *Nordic Journal of Music Therapy, 20*(3), 225-241.

Bailey, B. A., & Davidson, J. W. (2002). Adaptive characteristics of group singing: Perceptions from members of a choir for homeless men. *Musicae Scientiae, VI*(2), 221-256.

Bailey, B. A., & Davidson, J. W. (2003a). Amateur group singing as a therapeutic instrument. *Nordic Journal of Music Therapy, 12*(1), 18-33.

Bailey, B. A., & Davidson J. W. (2003b). Perceived holistic health effects of three levels of music participation. In R. Kopiez, A. C. Lehmann, I. Wohther, & C. Wolf (Eds.), *Proceedings of the 5th Triennial ESCOM Conference*, 8-13 September 2003, Hanover University of Music and Drama, Germany.

Bailey, B. A., & Davidson, J. W. (2005). Effects of group singing and performance for marginalized and middle-class singers. *Psychology of Music, 33*(3), 269-303.

Beck, R. J., Cesario, T. C., Yousefi, A., & Enamoto, H. (2000). Choral singing, performance perception, and immune system changes in salivary immunoglobulin A and cortisol. *Music Perception, 18*(1), 87-106.

Beck, R. J., Gottfried, T. L., Hall, D. J., Cisler, C. A., & Bozeman, K. W. (2006). Supporting the health of college solo singers: The relationship of positive emotions and stress to changes in salivary lgA and cortisol during singing. *Journal of Learning through the Arts: A Research Journal on Arts Integration in Schools and Communities, 2*(1), article 19.

Bigand, E., Vieillard, S., Madurell, F., Marozeau, J., & Dacquet, A. (2005). Multidimensional scaling of emotional responses to music: The effect of musical expertise and of the duration of the excerpts. *Cognition & Emotion, 19*(8), 1113-1139.

Blood, A. J., & Zatorre, R. J. (2001). Intensely pleasurable responses to music correlate with activity in brain regions implicated in reward and emotion. *Proceedings of the National Academy of Sciences, USA, 98*(20), 11818-11823.

Chlan, L. L. (1995). Psychophysiological responses of mechanically ventilated patients to music: A pilot study. *American Journal of Critical Care, 4*(3), 233-238.

Chong, H. J. (2010). Do we all enjoy singing? A content analysis of non-vocalists' attitudes towards singing. *The Arts in Psychotherapy, 37*(2), 120-124.

Clift, S. M. (2010). Singing for health: A musical remedy. *British Journal of Wellbeing, 1*(6), 14-16.

Clift, S. M., & Hancox, G. (2001). The perceived benefits of singing: Findings from preliminary surveys of a university college choral society. *Journal of the Royal Society for the Promotion of Health, 121*(4), 248-256.

Clift, S., Hancox, G., Staricoff, R., & Whitmore, C. (2008). *Singing and health: Summary of a systematic mapping and review of non-clinical research.* Sidney De Haan Research Centre for Arts and Health: Cantebury Christ

Church University.

Cohen, G. D., Perlstein, S., Chapline, J., Kelly, J., Firth, K. M., & Simmens, S. (2006). The impact of professionally conducted cultural programs on physical health, mental health, and social functioning of older adults. *The Gerontologist, 46*, 726-734.

Cohen, G. D., Perlstein, S., Chapline, J., Kelly, J., Firth, K. M., & Simmens, S. (2007). The impact of professionally conducted cultural programs on the physical health, mental health, and social functioning of older adults – 2-year results. *Journal of Aging, Humanities and the Arts, 1*, 5-22.

Csikszentmihalyi, M. (2002). *Flow*. London: Rider.

Davidson, J. W., & Faulkner, R. (2010). Meeting in music: The role of singing to harmonise carer and cared for. *Arts & Health: An International Journal of Research, Policy and Practice, 2*(2), 164-170.

Davidson, J. W., & Fedele, J. (2011). Investigating group singing activity with people with dementia and their caregivers: Problems and positive prospects. *Musicae Scientiae, 15*(3), 402-422.

Flood, M. (2006). Exploring the relationship between creativity, depression, and successful aging. *Activities, Adaptation, & Aging, 31*(1), 55-71.

Grape, C., Sandgren, M., Hansson, L. O., Ericson, M., & Theorell, T. (2003). Does singing promote well-being? An empirical study of professional and amateur singers during a singing lesson. *Integrative Physiological and Behavioral Sciences, 38*(1), 65-74.

Hills, P., & Argyle, M. (1998). Musical and religious experiences and their relationship to happiness. *Personality and Individual Differences, 25*, 91-102.

Juslin, P. N., & Laukka, P. (2003). Communication of emotions in vocal expression and music performance: Different channels, same code? *Psychological Bulletin, 129*(5), 770-814.

Kreutz, G., Bongard, S., Rohrmann, S., Grebe, D., Bastian, H. G., & Hodapp, V. (2004). Effects of choir singing or listening on secretory immunoglobulin A, cortisol and emotional state. *Journal of Behavioral Medicine, 27*(6), 623-635.

Kuhn, D. (2002). The effects of active and passive participation in musical activity on the immune system as measured by salivary immunoglobulin A (SigA). *Journal of Music Therapy, 39*(1), 30-39.

Lord, V. M., Cave, P., Hume, V. J., Flude, E. J., Evans, A., Kelly, J. L., Polkey, M. I., & Hopkinson, N. S. (2010). Singing teaching as a therapy for chronic respiratory disease: A randomized controlled trial and qualitative evaluation. *Pulmonary Medicine, 10*(41), 1-7.

McKinney, C., Antoni, M., Kumar, F., Tims, F., & McCabe, P. (1997). Effects of guided imagery and music (GIM) therapy on mood and cortisol in healthy adults. *Health Psychology, 16*(4), 390-400.

Oxford Dictionaries. (2013). Oxford Dictionaries. Retrieved from www.oxforddictionaries.com.

Ruud, E. (1997). Music and the quality of life. *Nordic Journal of Music Therapy, 6*(2), 86-97.

Ruud, E. (1998). *Music Therapy: Improvisation, Communication, and Culture*. Gilsum, NH: Barcelona Publishers.

Silber, L. (2005). Bars behind the bars: The impact of a women's prison choir on social harmony. *Music Education Research, 7*(2), 251-271.

Teater, B., & Baldwin, M. (2012). Singing for successful ageing: The perceived benefits of participating in the Golden Oldies community-arts programme. *British Journal of Social Work.* Published online first at http://bjsw.oxfordjournals.org/content/early/2012/07/02/bjsw.bcs095. doi: 10.1093/bjsw/bcs095.

Tuckman, B. (1965). Development sequence in small groups. *Psychological Bulletin, 63*(6), 384-399.

Unwin, M. M., Kenny, D. T., & Davis, P. J. (2002). The effects of group singing on mood. *Psychology of Music, 30,* 175-185.

Vink, A. (2001). Music and emotion. *Nordic Journal of Music Therapy, 10*(2), 144-158.

Chapter 5: Lost for Words: Drawing as a Visual Product and Process to Give Voice to Silenced Experiences

Lisa Hodge

"Engagement with the art form appears to simultaneously facilitate: the unearthing of unconscious material including memories, images and feelings; the production of an image or feelings which can be faced as acknowledged reality; and a way of communicating or speaking that reality" (Meekums, 1999, p.255).

Introduction

The central purpose of using drawings as a tool in research and therapy is to facilitate movement from internal to external expression, from silence to voice, from disconnection to connection, from disempowerment to empowerment. Drawings can give voice to that which has been unspeakable. The use of drawing as a resource to give disadvantaged groups a voice has been well established. For example, drawing has been utilised with children who are living in situations of political violence (Lykes, 1994), have chronic illness (Sartain, Clarke, & Heyman, 2000), have been exposed to domestic violence, physical and/or sexual abuse (Lefevre, 2004), to regulate emotions (Drake & Winnder, 2013), and whose parents are divorcing (Cordell & Bergman-Meador, 1991). The philosophy of art therapy more broadly, however, views drawing, and a variety of other art forms, as methods of expression available to everyone, regardless of age or abilities as everyone has the ability to be creative (Malchiodi, 2007). As such, it has also been utilised with women who are incarcerated (Merriam, 1998), living with post-traumatic stress disorder resulting from events such as war, violence, and natural disasters (Avrahami, 2006), sexual abuse survivors (Brooke, 1995), struggling with an eating disorder (Hinz, 2006), and diagnosed with borderline personality disorder (Eastwood, 2012). A container for powerful, potentially destructive emotions, drawing is a safe and acceptable way to release feelings such as anger and aggression.

The effects of sexual abuse and violence can be encoded within the body, mind, and psyche in ways that go beyond verbal thoughts; as such, the effects can be experienced as flashbacks and body memories (Anderson & Gold, 1998). Body memories, sometimes referred to as the "voice of the body" (Vigier, 1994, p. 236), are memories experienced through sensation rather than in the narrative form of ordinary memory (Haaken, 1996). Normal memories are automatically integrated into a personal narrative semantically and symbolically without conscious awareness of the process (Avrahami, 2006). In contrast, the nature of traumatic memories is dissociative; they are stored without symbolic and semantic components as visual sensory fragments, emotional attitudes, and fixed behaviours that are unchanged over time (Avrahami, 2006). Memories formed during bodily trauma are stored in the body and more easily accessed through physical expression (Mills & Daniluk, 2002). Visual materials can be used to generate rich description with regard to specific experiences by allowing participants to access remembered sensuous, emotional, spatial, and relational details (Del Busso, 2011). Drawing, as a product and a process, can enable people to share some of the effects of living in situations of abuse and violence as it facilitates self-expression and communication and allows the discharge of emotions connected to traumatic experiences.

Drawing can be a helpful tool in both research and therapy in accessing experiences that are simply beyond words. Within this chapter, the ways that drawings can provide opportunities to explore the multiplicity and complexity of the human experience are advanced (Guillemin, 2004). This chapter begins with an overview of how drawings are used to give participants a voice in research. Next, an exploration of how drawings are used in art therapy to promote healing among vulnerable populations is provided. I then review how drawings became an important source of information to the spoken word in my doctoral research on child sexual abuse and eating disorders. Using a case study as an example, I demonstrate how drawings created a path to one woman's feelings and helped her to reveal more than what may have been captured with only a verbal interview. The chapter concludes with suggestions for practitioners who seek to use drawing to gain further insight into the ways in which participants who have historically been oppressed make sense of their world.

To Find a Voice in Research: Breaking the Silence

Being silenced is a disempowering act. It can exacerbate traumatic experiences by fostering feelings of guilt and worthlessness. Pain is a private experience and describing it to others is difficult because it means translating feelings into words. Yet the ability to express emotions helps to protect the body from damaging internal stress that contributes to long-term health problems (Ullman, 2003). Thus, nonverbal forms of expression can provide an outlet for intense emotions, particularly visual representation.

Visual images are powerful forms of communication, and visual research has grown significantly, in part, due to an emphasis on the importance of culture in making sense of human experience (Pink, 2006). Visual research draws on a range of disciplines including sociology, anthropology, cultural studies, psychology, and art therapy (Prosser, 2007), and drawings as a method of inquiry have been commonly used in fields such as social anthropology (Collier & Collier, 1986). Visual artwork produced by research participants represents a powerful way to convey emotions (Leavy & Hesse-Biber, 2009). The use of drawing in research opens up multiple meanings (Leavy & Hesse-Biber, 2009), which are not only determined by the artist, but also the viewer and the context of viewing as they are experienced differently than text and sound.

Vulnerable populations are at risk of experiencing inequalities in health experiences and health outcomes and are generally the least heard within the context of research (Wilson & Neville, 2009). Research participants from vulnerable populations need to have their voices heard, yet research processes and outcomes can act to exacerbate vulnerability (Wilson & Neville, 2009). Moreover, society makes value judgments about the worth of this knowledge, which leads to further marginalisation of its members. For example, children's voices are silenced in society; they are often not privileged due to an explicit wish to protect their welfare. People who are not economically active, older members of society, ethnic minority groups, women, and people who are mentally ill, just to name a few are also silenced in society. Data collection methods that seek to give disadvantaged groups a voice require three prime characteristics: 1) they should provide a scope for individuals to be descriptive and analytical about their experiences; 2) they should match the communicative abilities of the individual; and 3) they should provide a mechanism through which the individual can express things they are afraid or unable to articulate (Sartain et al., 2000). One way that the representation of self or other aspects of personal biography can be discussed is through the exploration of participant's drawings (Sartain et al., 2000).

Case Example: Child Sexual Abuse

This case study presents Analiese[1], a 24-year old woman diagnosed with anorexia and dissociative identity disorder who was used in the production of child pornography from the age of two until she ran away from home as a teenager and became involved in the sex industry to survive. Her case was part of my doctoral dissertation, which sought to that examine women's understandings of the link between child sexual abuse and eating disorders.

Analiese asked me if her art diary could be used in the study as she found her experience difficult to talk about. The power of Analiese's drawings was the contextual and collaborative discussions that emerged as a result of them. Five interviews were conducted with Analiese over a 12-month period during which Analiese was asked about her drawings. These drawings became both a visual product and process, opening up multiple meanings determined not only by her, but also the viewer. After each interview, which was transcribed verbatim and analysed, I went back to Analiese and used my analysis to instigate further questions. Analiese critically reflected and expanded on her drawings and the emerging themes. Her interviews were fluid and their structure determined to a

---

[1] This is a pseudonym chosen by the participant and identifying factors have been changed for the purpose of confidentiality.

large extent by Analiese as she actively co-authored or co-constructed in this dialogical process.

Analiese said *Image 1* was a representation of one of her multiple personalities who she referred to as "Emily." In my analysis of *Image 1*, I paid particular attention to the social context of the image's production and effect. Analiese has depicted Emily's body without breasts, hips, or muscle development, and her hair is in pigtails, indicating a young child; yet she has drawn pubic hair surrounding cherries. This is symbolic of how Analiese's childhood, innocence, and virginity were ripped away from her at such a young age. Analiese has also drawn Emily with two sides: one dressed in ragged clothing with bare feet, indicating a child with low self-worth, and the other has fishnet stockings, a short dress, bright red lipstick, dyed hair, and handcuffs, which alludes to a prostitute. The viewer is confronted with memories of a childhood lost through imagery that includes a soft toy, a "REDSKIN" lolly, and Willy "Wonka" hat. These strongly contrast with the sophisticated prostitute. The difference is visualised in the physical separation of Emily's two sides. Here the pure and the fallen are juxtaposed, alluding to Analiese's self-construction as one of a wretched outcast. According to Nead (1990), visual images "have particular conditions of existence and are attended by special kinds of audience expectations which cannot be negated or collapsed into a reflection of other systems of representation" (p. 8). Visual culture does not absorb and transmit pre-formed ideology; it is not a neutral vehicle that expresses social meaning (Nead, 1990). Analiese's image tells the viewer how she saw herself morally and sexually. Through visual representation, the stereotype of the prostitute and the corruption of the fallen women is activated. Analiese's sense of self is constructed through the activating of the language of disease, evil, and sexual deviance.

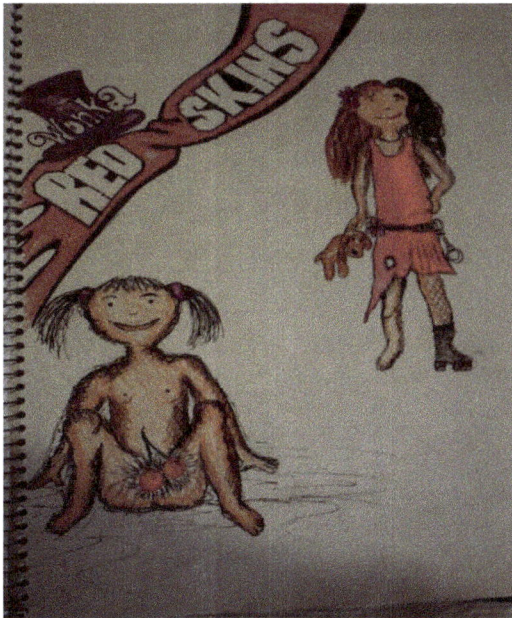

Image 1.

In *Image 2*, Analiese presents herself dressed in ragged clothing, which implies her sense of low self-worth and shame rather than her socioeconomic status as she comes from a middle class family with professional parents. Analiese uses colour in playful childhood imagery drawn purposefully at the edges of the picture to strongly contrast what she imagines childhood should be like with her actual experience—a childhood encapsulated by violence. Her lack of ears, nose, and mouth highlights her sense of being silenced and the powerlessness she feels within her situation. Analiese's wide-eyed expression illustrates her state of fear. The stitched cross in replacement of her mouth implies an inability to both speak and eat and thus a strong sense of silencing. Lack of limbs or body parts to interact with the environment are further indicative of helplessness and powerlessness (Gonick & Gold, 1992). The size of the clenched fists in comparison with Analiese's own self-representation emphasises the perpetrators' psychological and physical control.

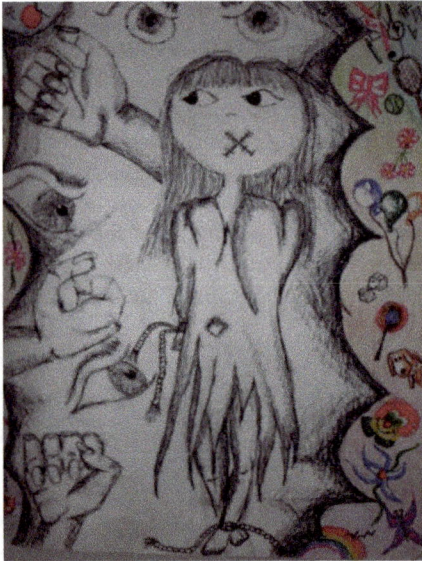

Image 2.

Analiese said *Image 2* was drawn while in the hospital four years ago and depicted her sense of feeling trapped and dominated by hands and fists. Analiese said having her lips stitched shut came up over and over again in her drawings. When I asked if the stitching of the mouth represented feeling unable to speak out about the abuse, Analiese said it was more about being trapped in the circumstances and silenced by society's hidden power structures. Analiese said an example was medicine and its power to label her with a mental illness, how this label defined her, and the stigma attached to that. She said the stitched mouth was also about knowing that she could not say anything because she was utterly terrified of being punched as she was constantly being monitored.

Both physical and psychological forces silenced Analiese. For her, the psychological force of being unable to speak and being tied up and trapped left her in a constant state of fear and doubting her ability to control other aspects of her life. Traumatic memories can be inaccessible to verbal memory, leaving trauma victims in a state of unspeakable terror. Yet drawing allows the trauma to "speak" in its own language–the visual form (Avrahami, 2006). To read further about the study, see: Hodge, L. (in press). How far to beautiful? Thinness, eating disorders, and sexual trauma. In S. McNamara (Ed.), *(Re)Possessing beauty: Politics, poetics, change*. Oxford, UK: Inter-Disciplinary Press.

Drawing as Therapy: Beyond Verbal Expression

Art heals because of the way people react to the artistic process and to the images produced (Hinz, 2006). According to Ramm (2005), drawing has the capacity to make "the invisible inner thought, vision, or experience visible" (p.66). Drawing is often used in counselling in conjunction with therapeutic techniques "to enhance therapy, move the individual to action, express thoughts, practice behaviours, and help the client to examine options" (Malchiodi, 2007, p. 228). Many social workers, mental health counsellors, marriage and family therapists, and psychologists use art therapy along with verbal counselling in their work (Malchiodi, 2007). Based on a process of creating visual images through drawing, painting, or clay modelling, art therapy evokes self-awareness (Merriam, 1998).

The ability of drawing to surface unspoken thoughts and feelings has long been accepted by art therapists (Kearney & Hyle, 2004; Malchiodi, 2007; Ramm, 2005). Practitioners have used this tool for many decades to facilitate expression because drawing "is not a linear process and need not obey the rules of language, such as syntax, grammar, logic, and correct spelling; it can express many complexities simultaneously" (Malchiodi, 2007, p.12). Through drawing or other art practices, practitioners can encourage clients to express what they cannot say with words. Drawing as therapy provides the opportunity to reconnect with disowned thoughts and feelings in a safe way and to contain them in the artwork; thus, this allows clients to gain distance from painful thoughts and feelings as well as to self-soothe (Merriam, 1998). Through their participation in drawing as a form of art therapy, clients do not have to reveal themselves verbally earlier than is comfortable (Hinz, 2006). Below, an overview of some of the applications for drawing in a therapeutic context is offered.

Children

Drawing is frequently used with children in therapeutic contexts. Children are generally comfortable with art as a way to communicate since they do not have extensive vocabulary for describing experiences (Malchiodi, 2007). "Drawing is a practical way of bringing children into an interview situation and of encouraging them to talk about themselves and their experiences" (Sartain et al., 2008, p. 917). Drawing can also generate questions. For example: What is happening here? What does it mean? How does it make me feel? (Sartain et al., 2000).

Drawing is an effective method in encouraging children to talk and reflect on their perceptions of their experiences. Children's drawings serve as an informative resource for capturing emotions and giving voice and agency to children (Kortesluoma, 2008). Research has shown that drawing facilitates a child's recall of painful memories, which otherwise would be difficult to share (Stafstrom, Rostasy, & Minster, 2002; Wesson & Salmon, 2001). Offering children an opportunity to draw can reveal their multi-level experiences and facilitate communication (Driessnack, 2005). In Lykes' (1994) study, problems encountered by Maya children of Guatemala in situations of ongoing war and state-sponsored terror were examined, he incorporated drawing, storytelling, collage, and dramatization in a group process. He found creative productions from the group, including drawings and collages, were a valuable tool to create a space and time in which children could express themselves, communicate experiences to others, and discharge emotions connected to previous traumatic experiences.

Walker, Myers-Bowman, and Myers-Walls' (2003) examined children's drawings and accompanying verbal statements of *peace* and *war* to investigate children's understandings of these concepts. They found that children were made aware of war through depictions of violence in the media, video games, movies, and the Internet more broadly. However, peace was not commonly understood, as it is not clearly defined in popular culture and the media. Thus, the children in his study needed help in understanding the concept of peace. Similarly, Goldner and Schart (2011) collected family drawings from 222 Israeli children to examine the relationship between children's attachment security and their personality and adjustment. They found that family drawings were an effective way to assess children's attachment representations and to identify children at risk for adjustment problems in schools. Drawings could be used to allow movement beyond adult conceptualisations and categories and provide an opportunity for children's authentic meanings to be recognised. Thus drawings can facilitate multiple understandings of the affective and cognitive lives of the children.

Women

Drawing can be used to facilitate communication of complex material and uncover troubling issues and conflicts. A nonverbal form of communication and expression, drawing can be important for highly traumatized women whose unspeakable feelings often lead to emotional withdrawal and isolation or the practice of destructive, tension-releasing activities (e.g., substance use, self-harm behaviours such as cutting, suicide attempts; Merriam, 2008). Child sexual abuse survivors frequently struggle with the effects of trauma into adulthood and may experience depression, posttraumatic stress disorder, anxiety, fear, and/or nightmares (Malchiodi, 2007). The trauma survivor can express dissociated feelings and memories symbolically in a work of art and may be able to express what was previously unspeakable. Many studies (see for example Eastwood, 2012; Lefevre, 2004; Merriam, 1998) suggest that the benefits of drawing with women who have been traumatised result from providing a protected environment for releasing tension, lowering defences, and gaining insight. Indeed, the value of drawing as a tool to recognise and undermine the power of oppression cannot be overstated. Eastwood (2012) notes:

> The complex nature of insidious trauma experienced by many women may be felt and yet not understood. Art making and the consequent

product is well equipped to expose, explore, and challenge the suppressed and disguised (p. 112).

An art image can offer distance from intense or overwhelming emotion so the feelings can be reflected upon and explored (Blatner, 1992). When working with clients who have experienced trauma, drawing can be used to reduce sources of shame, increase self-esteem, and offer the possibility of self-empowerment. In a study of how art therapy may be used to assist incarcerated women with histories of severe trauma to express their feelings, Merriam (1998) found drawing and other forms of artwork provided the women "with a voice when they [would] have otherwise lost their ability to verbalize their emotions because of trauma", and the process helped the woman to explore new ways of being (p.159). Lefevre's (2004) analysis of one woman's therapeutic journey, which took place over a two-year period, explicated the usefulness of metaphor and imagery in understanding, containing, and processing trauma provoked by familial sexual abuse.

Drawing may be beneficial for women who had been given the diagnosis of borderline personality disorder (BPD), which is often associated with complex trauma. Eastwood (2012) utilised drawing in group work for this client population and found that an understanding of trauma was achieved. "While nurturing the developed strategies towards empowerment, the client is able to understand their distress in a context in which they are not to blame [themselves] for past experiences, but can accept a personal responsibility in their process of change" (p. 112). Drawing can facilitate the exploration of alternative, less destructive ways of managing distress (Eastwood, 2012), allowing clients to begin the process of healing from past trauma.

Likewise, these benefits may also be realised with clients who have eating disorders. They are often filled with shame, which can impede them from openly discussing their experiences, or they may defensively guard their secrets. Thus, therapy sometimes proceeds with long periods of silence. Hinz (2006) argues drawings can be used to:

> contain and explain varied ideas, emotions, and conflicts in ways that words cannot. Art is an effective container for, and liberator from, the ambivalence that persons with eating disorders feel about recovery (p. 12).

This in turn may help clients process their feelings in a more constructive fashion and develop better coping skills. In sum, drawing offers a simple approach to working with traumatised women. Through visual expression, difficult thoughts and feelings can be expressed, explored, and processed, which facilitates healing and empowerment.

Health Applications

Drawing has been used in a number of different ways to explore health issues with children for therapeutic benefits. In one such study, children with cerebral palsy (CP) were asked to draw a picture of themselves walking. Results indicated that the size of the drawing along with the content (e.g., being in a building) were associated with walking ability (Chong, Mackey, Stott, & Broadbent, 2013). These drawings provide insight into how children with CP perceive their condition and may used to facilitate further exploration of their feelings (Chong et al., 2013). In another study, children were asked to create drawings of themselves engaged in some activity as they began a weight management program for children and families who are overweight. Results indicated that the majority of the children drew a picture where they were doing some type of physical activity (Walker, Caine-Bish, & Wait, 2009). Use of this approach could be beneficial when designing weight management programs for children to increase commitment to the plan (Walker et al., 2009).

The use of drawings has also been used to explore health issues amongst adults. For example, the drawings of 74 patients who had experienced a heart attack drew a picture of their heart just before they were released from the hospital. At a 3-month follow-up, researchers found that these drawings predicted recovery better than medical indicators (Broadbent, Petrie, Ellis, Ying & Gamble, 2004). That is, negative health beliefs, which were expressed in the drawings in the form of damage on the heart, predicted recovery. Thus, physicians could use these drawings as a way to discuss health and recovery beliefs following a heart attack (Broadbent et al., 2004). In a similar study, headache sufferers were asked to draw a picture of how their headache affected them. Content of the drawings was related to the type of suffering. For example, those participants who drew dark images had more emotional anguish (Broadbent, Niederhoffer, Hague, Corter, & Reynolds, 2009). Again, this would allow an additional way to evaluate the perception of pain and perspective on illness for individual patients (Broadbent et al., 2009). Drawing has also been found to be useful in helping patients to think about their disease (Lupus) in a way that is different from the medical view (Nowicka-Sauer, 2007). Through drawing, participants were able to concentrate on "feeling" and "experiencing" the disease (Nowicka-Sauer, 2007). These innovative health studies are illustrative of the many ways in which drawing can be used in practice to explore feelings, perceptions, health, pain, trauma, and illness.

Analysis of Drawings

Recent work within cultural studies provides useful ways of thinking about the analysis of visual imagery (Guillemin, 2004). Multiple conceptual frameworks exist from a range of different disciplines, yet there is no real widespread consensus about which methods should be used (Cross, Kabel, & Lysack, 2006). Knowles and Sweetman (2004) argue there are three paradigms of visual analysis: 1) realism, in which the visual image is regarded as evidence; 2) poststructuralist perspectives, through which images are used to help construct reality; and 3) semiotics, in which images are regarded as text which can be read and deconstructed into its component parts. Pink (2005) notes, "critical approaches to the interpretation of images has departed from the positivist 'truth-seeking' and objectifying approaches" (p. 31). Analysing visual data allows for an understanding of the participant's life through her/his drawings. In this sense "the accounts given and the interpretations made are then a result of a dialogic relationship between different positions" (Radley, 2010, p. 18).

Pulling from a poststructuralist perspective, drawings are conceptualised as a reflection of the culture from which they are part. An image's content is the "internal narrative" and the social relation in which the image is embedded at the time of viewing is the "external narrative" (Banks, 2001, p. 11–12). In order to look at the image but also look behind it, Rose's (2008) critical visual framework is an excellent resource for practitioners. According to Rose (2008), the interpretation of visual images exhibits three sites at which meanings of an image are made: the site of production of an image, the site of the image itself, and the site of the audience. Rose (2008) asserts that each of these sites has three different aspects to them—the compositionality, the technological, and the social modality of the image. The compositionality is best explained as the site of the image or object itself; that is, what is featured in the drawing and what it looks like, which includes the content, colour, and spatial organisation of the image. The technological is the site of production; that is, how an image is made and what materials are selected for the drawing. The social modality of the image is the site of its audiencing. What does the drawing mean within the given social, economic, and political context? What are the economic and political relations and practices that are embedded in an image through which it is viewed?

When analysing drawings in research or therapy, Guillemin's (2004) adaption of Rose's framework where the data comprises both the visual images and the participant's verbal descriptions of the image is another excellent alternative. It is important to ask the participant/client to describe her/his drawings. This is as an essential part of the method as it elicits the nature of the drawing and why s/he chose to draw that particular image. This process necessitates reflection on the part of the participant/client. It instigates critical reflections on how a participant's/client's drawing represents her/his experience and the significance of what s/he has drawn to her/his previous statements made during the interview.

Guillemin (2004) suggests asking participants a list of questions about the image itself. The following questions are adapted from Guillemin (2004):

- What is the context in which the image was produced?
- When was it made?
- What events preceded the drawing, in terms of the participant's condition?
- What were the relations between the drawer and the subject of the image?
- What is being shown?
- What are the components of the image?
- How are they arranged?
- What use is made of colour and what is its significance to the drawer?
- Is more than one interpretation of the image possible?

Merriam (1998) points out, "it is the focus on the image that makes art therapy distinct from verbal therapy and perhaps safer in that it is less intrusive" (p. 158). The image is experienced as tangible and produces a feeling of containment for potentially destructive emotions (Merriam, 1998). Asking about everything in a drawing mobilises new information and clarifies what the participant intended to express (Malchiodi, 2007). When working in a therapeutic context, the events, experiences, and interactions that precede the client's drawing act together to produce the understandings that are embedded in the drawings (Guillemin, 2004). Moreover, the process of helping the client to understand her/his own position can be therapeutic and healing (Eastwood, 2012).

Benefits and Potential Challenges

Despite the challenges this method may bring, drawing provides access to different meanings, interpretations, and themes that are not possible through other methods. Drawing affords a totally unique way for participants to tap into and express their feelings (Cross et al., 2006). It allows practitioners to enter the participants' experience more deeply. Drawing is a means to gain insight into a participant's world.

Drawing can be a useful source of information about many aspects of emotional illness (Nowicka-Sauer, 2007). It places the analytic lens upon the social intersection between "what is seen" and "what is felt" (Cross et al., 2006). Eastwood (2012) notes, "the complex nature of insidious trauma experienced by many women may be felt and yet not understood…art making and the consequent product is well equipped to expose, explore, and challenge the suppressed and disguised" (p. 112). Drawings enable participants to understand their distress in a context in which they are not to blame for past experiences. Thus, it is an empowering process. It facilitates the exploration of alternative, less destructive ways of managing distress from past trauma (Eastwood, 2012) and provides an alternative language with which to speak.

The use of drawing has some potential challenges. For researchers who use drawing and other visual data, they need to consider the limitations of using images as factual information given that "images are never transparent windows onto the world" (Rose, 2008, p.2). The interpretation of an image needs to be justified with an explicit methodology (Rose, 2008). When critically examining an image, we need to consider the image in terms of its cultural significance, social practices, and the power relations in which the image is embedded (Rose, 2008). Some methods of analysis are more methodical than others. Researchers and practitioners alike should consider if and how image analysis may be completed. Van Leeuwen and Jewitt (2008) point out:

> Some lay down very precise criteria for analysis, so that the impression may arise that visual analysis can be done "by rote," and described as kind of a recipe, a procedure to be followed step by step, without the need for any form of initiative, let alone inspiration (p. 8).

Moreover, this type of analysis entails thinking about how the images offer very particular visions of social categories such as class, race, gender, sexuality, and so on (Rose, 2008). It also involves practitioner's thinking about how it positions you, its viewer, in relation to it. A final issue to consider is the notion that drawings should be used alongside participants' explanations of them (Cross et al.,

2006). Interpretation is still limited to spoken or written words (Guillemin, 2004). Fundamentally, drawings are reduced to words in order to communicate about them.

Ethical Considerations

Practitioners and researchers should consider appropriate ways to achieve informed consent, anonymity/confidentiality, and dissemination when working with visual data. Ethical guidelines and codes of practice cover important principles, but visual data brings additional, potentially distinct, ethical conundrums. Image-based methods are collaborative and participatory, but can put participants at risk of being identified and misrepresented (Smith, 2008). Consideration of ethical issues is paramount when working with marginalised communities around sensitive issues. A participant's capacity to exercise autonomy and protect her/his own interests through informed consent can be impaired by vulnerability. Specific ethical issues need to be considered with people who are ill or have serious or life-limiting conditions (Lawton, 2001), who have limited intellectual abilities or mental health problems (Latvala & Vuokila-Oikkonen, 2000), who have cognitive impairment or decline that may be associated with age (Cameron, Lloyd, Kent, & Anderson, 2004) or marginality (Smith, 2008). According to Smith (2008), ethically appropriateness requires "awareness and sensitivity and is reflected in the degree of honesty and truthfulness in dealings with others" (p. 90).

A participant's written permission must be obtained before artwork is displayed outside the context of the agency; their informed consent should be gathered when presenting it within an agency at meetings, such as case conferences (Hinz, 2006). Participants' names might be covered, but if someone has a distinctive artistic style her/his identity may not be protected (Hinz, 2006). When giving informed consent to share artwork, clients must be reminded that their identity might be known from their artistic style (Hinz, 2006).

Participants (including children) need to understand the full implications of disclosure especially when drawings are displayed to the public. Parents must be asked for written consent for their children to participate. The information can be presented to the children in a simplified form and their assent can be asked for orally. During the process, the children's feelings and interests must be a priority. For a discussion on the legal issues concerning ownership and copyright of visual materials, including for example, paintings, collages, cartoons, sketches, graphs, diagrams, photographs, and films, see the *Recommended Readings* at the end of this chapter.

Tips for Practitioners

1. **What is your aim in using drawings in therapy?** Do you want the client to generate an image, which can be faced, witnessed, and appraised? Do you hope to unearth unconscious meaning? Are you using drawing for its containing and distancing properties? Is it the sense that the creation "speaks for" the survivor, either with or without the need for the usual use of language? Will you be using drawing for its ability to be

an effective vehicle for the meaningful expression of emotions and thoughts when words are not available? Have you considered that drawing can be used to express feelings in a tangible way? Will drawing be used as a tool to put ideas and images related to loss into a concrete form, which participants can then address?

2. **In thinking about the use of art as a therapeutic tool, will you need to consider factors related to age, gender, dexterity, mobility, or emotional well-being?** Will the drawings be used as a tool to reveal strengths, vulnerabilities, and weaknesses? Will drawing be a way to provide children with a possible starting point for helping them cope with difficulties? Are your participants physically able to complete the drawing task? Do your participants have the motor function needed to draw? Have you considered your participants' emotional state and how drawing may provide a safe outlet for emotions? Will it help your participants to understand the connection between their impulsive self-destructive acting out and what they are trying to avoid feeling? Have you discussed with your participant that the end product is something tangible that can provide a feeling of containment for your her/his fears and anxiety? Is it important for your participant's emotional state not to have to reveal her/him self verbally earlier than is comfortable?

3. **Have you considered that drawings are not culture-free?** When working with vulnerable populations, have you considered the ways you will reduce the risk of reinforcing negative or discriminatory points of view? Have you thought about the need to collaborate with colleagues who are intimately familiar with the culture of the participant? Cultural competence is needed when analysing drawings from diverse or distinct cultural backgrounds to recognise and interpret culture-specific symbols and related concepts (Walker, 2003). Practitioners need to be aware of the implications of imposing dominant cultural values on participants from non-dominant cultures as culturally sensitive art therapy has been lacking (Betts, 2013).

4. **How will you be analysing the drawings?** Will you be anticipating that the image will speak to you indirectly using metaphors? Will you be considering the drawing's formal design elements (e.g., colour, space) and recognizable content (e.g., figures, objects)? Will you be including verbal responses? Will both drawing and the description comprise the data? Have you considered how verbal descriptions can help to clarify content and provide data not necessarily presented visually? A participant's verbal descriptions can help prevent us from projecting our own values and ideas onto a drawing by making assumptions about what a participant is trying to communicate (Walker et al., 2003).

5. **Will you be using drawings to work with individuals, families, or groups?** Have you considered that drawing can shed light on children's perception of their families and parents? Can drawing create space for an interactional process of discovery? Have you considered that connection is critical to personal empowerment? Is it important for your participants to use drawing in a group setting because it has been found that this is beneficial for improving self-esteem? Will you be aiming to use drawing

to reduce feelings of powerlessness and disconnection from the self and others? If so, you might consider using drawing in group work. If considering using drawing in group work, will you screen for group member's basic ability to take care of self within the parameters of the group? Anderson and Gold (1998) point out "creative expression groups for women can be powerful ways of healing from violence and abuse" (p. 34). Nonverbal interventions within a group setting can facilitate containment, exploration, or expression of issues (Anderson & Gold, 1998).

6. **How will you manage participants who doubt in their drawing ability?** What if a participant feels unable to draw? Have you considered how artistic ability may inhibit or facilitate a participant's ability to articulate her/his understanding? Have you thought about how you will reassure your clients that art therapy does not depend on their ability to draw? Will you use gentle persuasion and phrases like "I don't expect you to be an artist" to elicit a drawing? Meaning making is often word based, and as such, some participants may experience difficulties in expressing themselves using images (Guillemin, 2004). However, Cross et al. (2006) argue when gentle persuasion is used, in nearly all instances, a drawing can be elicited.

7. **How will you analyse the visual data?** Will you use a framework? Will you have the person who created the image provide the interpretation? If you do the analysis, will you check your interpretation with that particular participant? How will you use this information?

8. **When working with vulnerable groups, have you planned for difficult emotional expression?** Are you trained to do this type of work? Do you have a co-facilitator? Are you aware of community resources and agencies that the participant may need to access?

9. **Can drawing be used adjunctively with your current practice to facilitate emotional expression and personal growth or change?** Drawing can be incorporated into individual and group counselling as a short intervention or something that occurs with some regularity throughout the work. Adding visual pieces to talk-based work has the potential to enhance the process.

10. **Have you considered a public display of visual information to raise community awareness about an important issue?** This must be fully discussed and explored with participants to determine if they want their work to be shown. If they are interested in the idea, then they should retain control over what is shown. Drawing can be a powerful way to highlight difficult or complex personal and social issues. Public displays and forums may help to raise awareness about critical issues such as abuse and violence.

Recommended Readings and Resources

Buchalter, Susan I. (2009). *Art therapy techniques and applications.* London: Jessica Kingsley.

Clark, A., Prosser, J., & Wiles, R. (2010). Ethical issues in image-based Research. *Arts & Health: An International Journal for Research, Policy and Practice, 2*(1), 81-93.

Malchiodi, C. A. (2012). *Handbook of art therapy.* New York: Guilford Press.

Pink, S. (2007). *Doing visual ethnography* (2nd ed.). London: Sage.

Rubin, J. A. (2005). *Child art therapy.* Hoboken, NJ: John Wiley.

References

Anderson, L., & Gold, K. (1998). Creative connections: The healing power of women's art and craft work. *Women & Therapy, 21*(4), 15-36.

Avrahami, D. (2006). Visual art therapy's unique contribution in the treatment of post-traumatic stress disorders. *Journal of Trauma & Dissociation, 6*(4), 5-38.

Banks, M. (2001). *Visual methods in social research.* London: Sage.

Betts, D. (2013). A review of the principles for culturally appropriate art therapy assessment tools. *Art Therapy: Journal of the American Art Therapy Association, 30*(3), 98-106.

Blatner, A. (1992). Theoretical principles underlying creative arts therapies. *The Arts in Psychotherapy, 18,* 405–409.

Brooke, S. L. (1995). Art therapy: An approach to working with sexual abuse survivors. *The Arts in Psychotherapy, 22*(5), 447-466.

Brown, L. S. (2010). *Feminist therapy.* Washington, DC: American Psychological Association.

Broadbent, E., Niederhoffer, K., Hague, T., Corter, A., & Reynolds, L. (2009). Headache sufferers' drawings reflect distress, disability and illness perceptions. *Journal of Psychosomatic Research, 66,* 465-470.

Broadbent, E., Petrie, K. J., Ellis, C. J., Ying, J., & Gamble, G. (2004). A picture of health—myocardial infarction patients' drawings of their hearts and subsequent disability: A longitudinal study. *Journal of Psychosomatic Research, 57,* 583-587.

Cameron, A., Lloyd, L., Kent, N., & Anderson, P. (2004). Researching end of life in old age: Ethical challenges. In M. Smyth & E. Williamson (Eds.), *Researchers and their "subjects": Ethics, power, knowledge and consent* (pp. 105–117). Bristol: Policy Press.

Chong, J., Mackey, A. H., Stott, N. S., & Broadbent, E. (2013). Walking drawings and walking ability in children with cerebral palsy. *Health Psychology, 32*(6), 710-713.

Collier, J., & Collier, M. (1986). *Visual anthropology: Photography as a research method.* Albuquerque, New Mexico: University of New Mexico Press.

Cordell, A. S., & Bergman-Meador, B. (1991). The use of drawings in group intervention for children of divorce. *Journal of Divorce and Remarriage, 17*(1/2), 139-155.

Cross, K., Kabel, A., & Lysack, C. (2006). Images of self and spinal cord injury: Exploring drawing as a visual method in disability research, *Visual Studies, 21*(2) 183-193.

Del Busso, L. (2011). Using photographs to explore the embodiment of pleasure in everyday life. In P. Reavey (Ed.), *Visual methods in psychology: Using and interpreting images in qualitative research* (Ch. 4). London: Routledge.

Drake, J. E., & Winner, E. (2013). How children use drawing to regulate their emotions. *Cognition and Emotion, 27*(3), 512-520.

Driessnack, M. (2005). Children's drawings as facilitators of communication: A meta-analysis. *Journal of Pediatric Nursing*, 20(6), 415–23.

Eastwood, C. (2012). Art therapy with women with borderline personality disorder: A feminist perspective. *International Journal of Art Therapy: Formerly Inscape, 17*(3), 98-114.

Goldner, L., & Scharf, M. (2011). Children's family drawings: A study of attachment, personality, and adjustment. *Art Therapy: Journal of the American Art Therapy Association, 28*(1), 11-18.

Gonick, R. S., & Gold, M. (1992). Fragile attachments: Expressive arts therapy with children in foster care. *The Arts in Psychotherapy, 18,* 433-440.

Guillemin, M. (2004). Understanding illness: Using drawings as a research method. *Qualitative Health Research, 14*(2), 272-289.

Haaken, J. (1996). The recovery of memory, fantasy, and desire: Feminist approaches to sexual abuse and psychic trauma. *Signs, 21*(4), 1069-1094.

Hinz, L. D. (2006). *Drawing from within: Using art to treat eating disorders.* London: Jessica Kingsley.

Kearney, K. S., & Hyle, A. E. (2004). Drawing out emotions: The use of participant-produced drawings in qualitative inquiry. *Qualitative Research, 4,* 361-382.

Knowles, C., & Sweetman, P. (2004). *Picturing the social landscape: Visual methods and the sociological imagination.* London: Routledge.

Kortesluoma, R. L., Punamäki, R. L., & Nikkonen, M. (2008). Hospitalized children drawing their pain: The contents and cognitive and emotional characteristics of pain drawings. *Journal of Child Health Care, 12*(4), 284-300.

Latvala, E., & Vuokila-Oikkonen, P. (2000). Videotaped recording as a method of participant observation in psychiatric nursing research. *Journal of Advanced Nursing, 31*(5), 1252–1257.

Lawton, J. (2001). Gaining and maintaining informed consent: Ethical concerns raised in a study of dying patients. *Qualitative Health Research, 11,* 69–73.

Leavy, P. (2009). *Method meets art: Arts-based research practice.* New York: Guilford.

Leavy, P., & Hesse-Biber, S. N. (Eds.). (2009). *Handbook of emergent methods.* New York: Guilford Press.

Lefevre, M. (2004). Finding the key: Containing and processing traumatic sexual abuse. *The Arts in Psychotherapy, 31,* 137-152.

Lykes, M. B. (1994). Terror, silencing and children: International, multidisciplinary collaboration with Guatemalan Maya communities. *Social Science & Medicine, 38*(4), 543-552.

Malchiodi, C. A. (2007). *The art therapy source book.* New York: McGraw-Hill.

Meekums, B. (1999). A creative model for recovery from child sexual abuse trauma. *The Arts in Psychotherapy, 26*(4), 247–259.

Merriam, B. (1998). To find a voice: Art therapy in a women's prison. *Women & Therapy, 21*(1), 157-171.

Mills, L., & Daniluk, J. C. (2002). Her body speaks: The experience of dance therapy for women survivors of child sexual abuse. *Journal of Counseling & Development, 80*, 77-85.

Nead, L. (1990). *Myths of sexuality: Representations of women in Victorian Britain*. United Kingdom: Blackwell.

Nowicka-Sauer, K. (2007). Patients' perspective: Lupus in patients' drawings. *Clinical Rheumatology*, 26, 1523-1525.

Pink, S. (2005). *The future of visual anthropology: Engaging the senses*. New York: Routledge.

Pink, S. (2006). *Doing visual ethnography: Images, media and representation in research* (2nd ed.). London: Sage.

Prosser, J. (2007). Visual methods and the visual culture of schools. *Visual Studies, 22*(1), 13-30.

Radley, A. (2010). What people do with pictures. *Visual Studies, 25*(3), 268-279.

Ramm, A. (2005). What is drawing? Bringing the art into art therapy. *International Journal of Art Therapy: Formerly Inscape, 12*(2), 63-77.

Reavey, P. (Ed.). (2011). *Visual methods in psychology: Using and interpreting images in qualitative research*. New York: Routledge.

Rose, G. (2008). *Visual methodologies: An introduction to the interpretation of visual materials* (2nd ed.). London: Sage.

Sartain, S. A., Clarke, C. L., & Heyman, R. (2000). Hearing the voices of children with chronic illness. *Journal of Advanced Nursing, 32*(4), 913-921.

Stafstrom, C. E., Rostasy, K., & Minster, A. (2002). The usefulness of children's drawings in the diagnosis of headache. *Pediatrics, 109*(3), 460–72.

Smith, L. (2008). How ethical is ethical research? Recruiting marginalised, vulnerable groups into health services research. *Journal of Advanced Nursing, 62*(2), 248–257.

Ullman, S. (2003). Social reactions to child sexual abuse disclosures: A critical review. *Journal of Child Sexual Abuse, 12*(1), 89-121.

Van Leeuwen, T., & Jewitt, C. (Eds.). (2008). *The handbook of visual analysis*. London: Sage.

Vigier, R. (1994). *Gestures of genius: Women, dance and the body*. Stratford, Ontario: Mercury Press.

Walker, K., Caine-Bish, N., & Wait, S. (2009). "I like to jump on my trampoline": An analysis of drawings from 8-to12-year-old children beginning a weight-management program. *Qualitative Health Research, 19*(7), 907-917.

Walker, K., Myers-Bowman, K. S., & Myers-Walls, J. A. (2003). Understanding war, visualizing peace: Children draw what they know. *Art Therapy: Journal of the American Art Therapy Association, 20*(4), 191-200.

Wesson, M., & Salmon, K. (2001). Drawing and showing: Helping children to report emotionally laden events. *Applied Cognitive Psychology, 15*(3), 301–320.

Wilson, D., & Neville, S. (2009). Culturally safe research with vulnerable populations. *Contemporary Nurse, 33*(1), 69-79.

Chapter 6: Connecting through Clay: Sculpting Tactile Expressions of Deep Held Emotions

Fiona Buchanan

Introduction

Sculpture represents a unique form of creative expression in that the medium can embody and make solid interpretations of emotions. It can be an outlet for memories and lead to insightful meaning. Clay moulding, in particular, can be a powerful way for people to express feelings through a tactile connection. In the process of working with clay, verbal communication can be facilitated and a cathartic release may occur; one that cannot be accessed through words alone. The emotional work that transpires through the process of using clay acts to connect the individual both with her/his inner-self and also with the practitioner and other participants during group work. Within this safe space, deep connections can be made with supportive others.

In this chapter, the properties of clay work in therapy, group work, and community are described. The need for clay work to be positioned in a setting of safety is explained, and the processes of this work are described. An example of using clay with women who have endured domestic abuse is given to illustrate how clay modelling can uncover new knowledge while enabling participants to access feelings of emancipation, connection, and empowerment. Ethical considerations and practicalities of working with clay are also outlined.

The Arts and Emotions

Artwork, in general, can enable increased insight as well as an opportunity for reflection (Waller, 1992). Visual art helps people to access their inner life and to then evaluate that representation to safely witness past experiences, which may have been confined to the subconscious in a bid for self-protection. McNiff (2011) acknowledges "the personal and even intimate qualities of artistic inquiry," which cues us to the fact that art is a deep and meaningful method of self-expression (p. 364). Elsewhere, Simons and McCormack (2007) refer to art as an aid to individuals "revealing insights they cannot articulate in words" (p.296).

Sometimes art goes beyond words, and during the process of creating, people open up and become more articulate. Firstly, creating visual representations gives voice to the inner world of the maker, and secondly, the creator can then interpret her/his art to communicate thoughts and feelings to others.

There is something in the process of making art that frees emotions that have been locked inside. Art is particularly relevant to trauma because it "involves the brain's hemispheres in accessing memories and processing emotions" (Talwar, 2007, p. 26). Clay work can be particularly powerful in allowing survivors of abuse to achieve catharsis and release from shame and guilt. Perhaps this is because clay work allows people not only to see, but also feel and handle the representations of their inner worlds. Because the hands are in direct contact with clay, memories and insights previously unacknowledged are brought to mind (Talwar, 2007). Once such thoughts and emotions are made visible to the clay maker, they are there to be deliberated, touched, and deconstructed. As has been noted:

> ...moulding clay can be a powerful way to help people express these feelings through tactile involvement at a somatic level, as well as to facilitate verbal communication and cathartic release and reveal unconscious materials and symbols that cannot be expressed through words (Stuckey & Nobel, 2010, p.4)

Sculpting can bring balance to one's life, whether by viewing great works of art such as those by Rodin, Moore, and Lucchesi, sculpting one's own creations, or witnessing the creations of others who are working to express their inner thoughts. Sholt and Garron (2006) define clay work as "the process of handling, manipulating and sculpting clay and the products of these activities" (p. 66). Both the process and the end product are important. Whatever the skill level, the end result is visual, tactile, and three-dimensional. All three qualities combine to affect feelings. Visually, the made object is formed to be as simple or complex as the maker wishes. The tactile experience is both intense and powerful (Sholt & Garron, 2006). There is no pen or brush to afford distance from the material; the shape is formed directly in connection with the emotional self. Clay effectively embodies and makes solid an interpretation of internal emotions that are often the conduit for memories and insightful meaning. In working directly with the material, which is soft, squidgy, and malleable, there is direct communication with the actual clay, moving, moulding, and having mastery over shape and texture. This is powerful and empowering; it is not predetermined, and all is in the maker's control. There is also a sense of creating something from nothing; that is, nothing but a lump of mud (Sholt & Garron, 2006). From nothing, there are infinite possibilities to demonstrate uniqueness and connect with others through sharing a visual, tactile, and multidimensional mode of self-expression.

Working with clay, the maker has control over both form and texture. Form can be infinitely changed, and the remoulding can bring new thoughts and emotions to the clay model. This creates multiple visual perspectives, which can each represent different facets of emotionally charged insights. Also, texture can be introduced to form a range of diverse surfaces from bumpy, rutted, and jagged to smooth, even, and rounded. In this way, surfaces can be used to present metaphors for feelings. Through form and texture, loss and suffering can be embodied and sadness and anger expressed. Joy might be embedded symbolically and even comfort can be expressed through flowing shapes. Another useful aspect of clay work is that once a negative experience or emotion has been embodied, flattening, squashing, and punching can physically destroy it. Residual anger can be safely released and the model maker has the ability to destroy and reconstruct with the same materials, which enables a sense of control and empowerment over the process.

The work of clay moulding involves emersion in the process of connecting physically and emotionally. It involves letting go of the conscious and letting the hands create meaning. It is hard emotional work, although, surprisingly the process itself is unemotional. It is as if, while working with clay, emotions are being transferred into the material. For people who have not immersed themselves in clay work, the process can be slightly daunting, but if they are encouraged to get past the mechanics by literally "feeling" their way intuitively, the end result can be a sense of wonder. The processing can uncover new perspectives, which then lead to a sense of peace and well-being. Fresh insights into the inner self that allow resolution of troubling feelings are accessed and can enable recognition of heartfelt emotions leading to compassion for self and pride in one's ability to survive.

Emotions relate to touch (Dickson-Swift James, Kippen, & Liamputtong, 2009), and clay is a tactile medium which can facilitate the connection between emotions and cognition. In research aiming to investigate the effect of clay on emotions, a randomised control trial was undertaken to discover if clay work could reduce negative moods (Kimport & Robbins, 2012). In this study, 102 people recruited from a university campus were allocated to one of three groups. The first group was given stress balls, the second group was given balls of clay and instructions to make a pot, and the third was given balls of clay with no instructions. Each participant worked in isolation. Participants rated their feelings of "tension, depression, fatigue, confusion, anger, and vigor" prior to the intervention and again afterwards (Kimport & Robbins, 2012, p.76). Results showed that "clay work has unique properties for emotional expression and regulation that go beyond the simple manipulation of an object" (Kimport & Robbins, 2012, p.77). The group with the instructions to make a pot was found to have slightly better effects, and this led the authors to hypothesis that a task that led to a completed object would better suit art therapy interventions. While negative emotions were introduced superficially in a simulated laboratory setting, which is quite different from using clay to access deeply held emotions, this study offers some evidence for the use of clay work and the reduction of negative mood states.

Using Clay in Therapy

As noted, clay is not solely an introspective medium; clay can also provide a means of communicating to others about lived experiences. A study, which investigated the interaction between clay and ideas, thoughts, and feelings found that the "dialogue" between the maker and the clay could help therapists and clients to share meanings (Bar-on, 2007). Twenty "non-artist" students were recruited from an Israeli University, and visual and verbal data from two sessions with each student was thematically analysed. In the first session, students worked with the clay in a structured setting with the instruction "through the clay tell us about yourself" (Bar-on, 2007, p. 5). Semi-structured interviews were used to access spontaneous reflections. After 1-2 weeks, a second session was organised where videotapes, taken of the individuals working with the clay during the earlier sessions, were viewed and participants were asked about their experiences. Bar-on (2007) describes clay work and reflection as "thinking and doing in two languages" and describes working with clay as an educational experience, which generates ideas for problem solving (p. 16).

However, if working therapeutically with clients, an important component of clay work is also the feelings work evoked by thinking and doing in this alternative language. Practitioners are privileged to witness and work with clients' insights as they access emotions through their expressive clay work as such work can deepen the relationships with clients. As clients share deeply held feelings, both therapist and client are able to better understand, reach for meaning, and acknowledge the strengths and strategies that are employed to ensure survival. Self-recognition of strategies for survival is important because clients too often see themselves as powerless and are perceived by others as victims when, in fact, they have used their agency to endure and withstand adversity. Sometimes negative emotions generated by destructive beliefs can hold clients back from reaching their full potential. In a study of individuals undergoing therapy, Henley (2002) found that clay work allows clients to safely express and release negative emotions such as anger and aggression. This study suggests that expression through clay work can allow previously unrealised emotions to surface and a new sense of well-being to be uncovered. Thus, the use of clay during the therapeutic process may provide additional insights and growth for the client.

Using Clay in Group Work

Connecting with others through clay work is not, however, confined to the privacy of a therapist's office. Clay is also renowned as a medium which aids expressive communication in group work (Carozza & Heirsteiner, 1982). With groups of adult survivors of sexual abuse, clay work has been found to provide catharsis and a means to empowerment. A qualitative study evaluated two clay therapy groups with five survivors in each group. Using follow-up questionnaires at three and six months, this study found that participants felt significantly better about themselves following the groups and that the sense of well-being was sustained over a six-month period (Anderson, 1995). In another study, 41 patients with Parkinson's disease and their caregivers were asked to work with balls of clay and then complete a questionnaire about their experience. This study found that working with clay evoked a positive emotional response in most participants, and the researchers recommended that clay be used in groups to reduce somatic symptoms and emotional distress for both patients and caregivers (Elki-Abuhoff, Goldblatt, Gaydos, & Corrato, 2011).

Furthermore, within feminist research, clay work has been utilised to achieve greater understandings of emotional issues. A qualitative study by Huss (2007) employed women's self-explanations of their drawings and clay work to connect with the experiences of impoverished Bedouin women. This study found that the dialogues between women, which occurred while they focused on drawing and clay work, helped to develop empathy among group participants. In light of this, Huss (2007) described painting and clay work in groups as "a clarifying and cognitive act" rather than cathartic expression (p. 979). However, it is possible that clay work can be used as a means of both expressing feelings and clarifying thoughts as the two are not mutually exclusive. In another feminist study, Walsh (2006) explored experiences of teachers' fear and pain and incorporated various art mediums to access feelings and mood. Findings suggest that the process of working with clay and other materials lead to the emergence of differing interpretations and perspectives. Although Walsh (2006) describes art work as "a trigger for words rather than a central activity" (p. 963), it could also be suggested that art provides a process and an end product of creation, which helps participants make meaning.

The impact of violence against women is often described in terms of "mental health" with a focus on the pathological effects of violence against women who have been abused by others. It is not disputed that the degradation, humiliation, and manipulative tactics of abusers can adversely affect mental health; however, domestic violence firstly constitutes an assault on physical safety and emotional well-being. When women recall the effects of domestic abuse, child sexual abuse, rape, and sexual assault, it is often with remembered fear and with feelings of shame, self-blame, and guilt. These feelings are exacerbated by societal views, which perceive victims of such abuse as either responsible for their own victimisation or damaged for life. Treating survivors as mentally unwell does not effectively address emotional suffering or allow survivors to challenge the beliefs that underpin such distress. In addition, acquiring a psychiatric label that describes the effects of abuse as an illness is not empowering. Emotions resulting from domestic abuse, child sexual assault, rape, and sexual abuse are not mental health issues; they are understandable emotional reactions that may, if unattended, lead to mental health issues (Herman, 1992). Whether or not gendered abuse leads to mental health problems, being abused can inhibit emotional well-being and silence the voices of women who have endured unspeakable assaults. Empowerment comes from being enabled to give voice to these experiences and their effects. This is where clay can be a powerful tool as it allows the unspeakable to be expressed.

For survivors of abuse, the process of having control of a malleable medium allows feelings to be accessed, embodied, and expressed in a three-dimensional form, which can then be described and communicated. In a study that sought to evaluate the efficacy of five different art materials, the three-dimensional aspect of clay work and the ability to ascribe meaning to a tangible article resulted in participants placing a high value on the therapeutic use of clay. The researchers who undertook this study sum up participants views by concluding:

> Clay is experienced as clean and more controllable, enabling a sense of self efficacy and security...with clay one can work with either rough or light, small or large movements, enabling the expression of different emotions (Snir & Regev, 2012, p. 99).

Moreover, empowerment is enabled through accessing understanding and appreciation of self and being able to convey heartfelt emotions so that others may understand. When women who have survived abuse are brought together in therapeutic groups, clay work can be a powerful pathway to finding common ground. Through sharing interpretations of their clay work, individuals can collaborate in a process of mutual empowerment that can transform their collective lives. By accessing the capacity to name, reflect, and act the shame, the silencing effects of abuse can be confronted. Through working with clay in survivor groups, women can collectively name the experiences that result in emotional turmoil, reflect on shared emotions, and act to support each other to overcome the limiting effects of abuse.

Case Example: Researching Mother/Baby Relationships through Clay Work

In a community based research study, 16 women who had left abusive partners at least one year prior to the study participated in focus groups about experiences of forming mother/baby relationships while enduring domestic violence. The aim of the groups was to help women locate emotional experiences and process sensitive issues. Initial interviews were held in the women's homes, then two sets of focus groups were organised. During interviews and the first focus groups, supportive relationships with the participants were established. In the first focus group, participants also worked together on a collage about mothering in domestic violence so that they became comfortable with a hands-on method of communication. Clay work was introduced in the second focus groups once trust and safety were established. In this session, each woman created an abstract clay model of her experience of building a relationship with her baby while enduring domestic violence. The clay models were photographed and accompanied by the words that each woman used to describe her clay model. Before ending the final focus group session, each woman was asked to create another clay model to represent hopes for the future of her relationship with her child. This task was important as it enabled women to visualise a future with hope rather than to leave the study focused on difficult times.

The women's descriptions of their clay models were an important focus of analysis as the process of clay work brought deeply held emotional insights to the research. The clay works represented here are chosen because they illustrate two diverse ways that women used the clay to demonstrate feelings. The models and the women's words exemplify heartfelt recollections that were accessed through the clay work. For example, Kate represented her growing understanding of the circumstances, which led to her withdrawing emotionally.

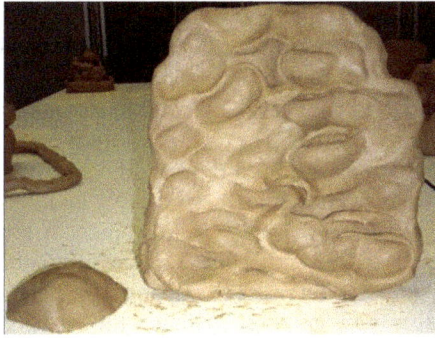

Image 1.

Kate: ...I have nothing because there is this big wall and this barrier that's stopped us from having a relationship, and it's not anything specific, but it's everything, it's me withdrawing. To protect my children but having to withdraw from them and having to be numb and not feel anything including them, in order to be able to protect them (very distressed-taking deep breaths). I'm past the tears now I'm just fucking angry (said emphatically).

Tanya's model illustrated the chaos that she felt when she was trying to care for her baby while enduring violence.

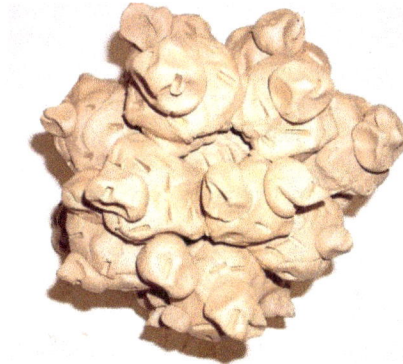

Image 2.

Tanya: ...holes in everything, emotionally, mentally...emotion flooding out and clinging to the side of me and all of this on top is just all the other stuff of life, the big and the small just issues and that's all got holes in it as well and it's not particularly orderly and it's complicated and there's just a big mess and it's all on my shoulders...(crying).

While describing their clay models women expressed anger, grief, tenderness, pride, hurt, and joy; however, the women also felt that although emotional revisiting had been draining, they had found that expressing themselves through clay modelling was cathartic. Empowerment came from revealing deeply held thoughts and finding that through clay work others understood these experiences. Clay modelling embodied their struggles to relate to their babies and made visible their strengths and efforts to protect their babies. Through describing their clay work, the women connected with each other and found empowerment through the relationships that were formed. The findings from the research uncovered important insights that are used to inform practitioners who work to enhance the life experiences of women and children who have endured domestic violence. Furthermore, the clay work produced by the women in their focus groups has connected with practitioners and policy makers attending Australian and international presentations of the research. By including photographs of the work produced in this research in presentations, the insights of women who experienced domestic violence while raising their babies underpins the author's spoken words and conveys meaning and emotions in ways that are more powerful than works alone can ever do (for a full account of the research see Buchanan, Power, & Verity, 2013).

Clay and Play

The effect of using clay work to address emotions and gain clarity necessitates experience of the process, which goes beyond the explicable and cognitive. It is in some way primal. Indeed, another dimension of clay work is that it has the ability to connect with early recollections of playing in the mud as small children. There is delight and pleasure for adults to be given permission to get messy. Participants who are rather anxious and describe themselves as "not arty" often begin to handle the clay tentatively. They may quickly recall memories of mud pies, plasticine, and play-do. Within the comfort of playing, the expectations of performance are reduced and emotional work begins. Sometimes the first emotion to be accessed is delight. Perhaps recalling the ease with which children express emotions helps participants to express their emotional selves through clay. For example, in group work sessions with participants who suffer from depression and anxiety, spending a session making a clay representation of a happy time from childhood can help participants to connect with the joy and delight of childhood and share memories that counter distress and despair. Perhaps the idea of child's play within a safe space in the company of trusted others enables participants to connect with and reveal their inner world. Whatever the reason, clay can be a powerful and empowering medium in group work.

In addition to the previously discussed qualities of clay, it clay can also be a useful medium for connecting with children. For them, clay work creates a fun and safe environment where the focus on verbalising experiences and troubles is removed. As part of building relationships, asking children to use the clay to create a world where they would like to live can open the door to imagination, hope, and connection while engaged in constructive play. Children find that clay can be moulded easily, it is wonderfully messy, and models can be constructed, deconstructed, and reformed. If children want to express angry feelings they can do this safely through pounding, smashing, or destroying images that they do not want in their world. For children with limited verbal capacity, clay gives access to an alternative way of communicating by offering another language where wishes, feelings, and fears can be expressed (Waller, 2006).

Community Work and Clay

One of the elements of clay work that differentiates it from two-dimensional art forms is that it can be viewed from many sides. Both the maker and the viewer can see different facets of the issues that are represented. Clay offers a holistic representation that simultaneously allows access to different aspects of the whole. In this way, clay can be shaped to represent the complexity of perceptions, feelings, and thoughts that encompass the issue under scrutiny. Artwork in the community helps members to "name and understand their realities, identify their needs and strengths, and transform their lives" (Golub, 2005, p.17). Although clay work is an intensely introspective activity when it is used in this manner, it can be a way to represent self to others and to connect with their experiences. Through the process of the maker showing and describing their creation, feelings, inner thoughts, and experiences may resonate with others and lead to a sense of solidarity. In a community where others have endured similar experiences, such a powerful connection can mean an end to isolation and enable "private and social transformation" (Golub, 2005, p. 21). Golub (2005) connects art as a process with Freire's (1970) pursuit of community empowerment. While Golub's work is primarily with oppressed communities throughout the world, any community development initiative which seeks to create a safe space by helping members use self-expression to find a common purpose could make use of clay. For example, community development that seeks to create a neighbourhood that embraces difference could begin with visioning "tolerance" through clay models to prompt discussion and garner ideas.

Benefits and Potential Challenges

One of the primary benefits of clay is that it is very versatile. It can be used with individuals, groups, and communities and for a variety of different goals. Clay can also be used with clients and participants from all age groups. Physical limitations and cognitive capacity do not restrict participation. Secondly, clay allows for the expression of complex emotional experiences, which may lead to additional insights and evolutions for the maker. Thirdly, clay work is an empowering approach to practice. Regardless of the primary goal, a practitioner hopes that the client will achieve the ability to control the clay form and express different emotions, which leads to a sense of self-efficacy and an ability to connect with others. Finally, clay is inexpensive. Unlike some art mediums, which require considerable initial outlay and continuing replenishment as materials are used, clay is cheap, recyclable after use, and with minimum preparation, it can be stored indefinitely.

However, there are two primary challenges with using clay work in practice. Firstly, clients and group member who are unfamiliar with clay may feel anxious and have a sense of trepidation about their ability to work with an unknown medium. Secondly, the emotional turmoil that can be raised through clay work's ability to evoke emotions needs to be anticipated. Both of these issues can be addressed through the building of trusting relationships with clients and between group participants to create a safe space to explore a new way of communication and emotional expression.

Ethical Considerations

When introducing clay into practice, there is a need to warn clients, group participants, and co-workers that clay may lead them to unexpected emotions and raise previously unexplored memories. For example, the author co-facilitated a child sexual survivors group once with a clinical psychologist who worked from a cognitive behavioural perspective. During the group session with clay, the psychologist opened herself to the experience of feeling through clay. Although the author had explained the process and the likely outcomes, the co-facilitator was overwhelmed by her ability to see herself and her own past mirrored in a way that conventional approaches to therapy did not reveal.

With the powerful and sometimes unexpected results of working with clay, there is a need to establish safety and trust with those who are involved. It is important to prepare for clay work so that clients in therapy and participants in group work feel safe and permitted to express emotions. Feeling safe can take time to develop; it may need to evolve over several individual or group sessions. Creating safety is skilled work involving thoughtful planning and intuitive practice on the part of the practitioner. For example, the author once overlooked an important element of establishing rapport when she was invited to facilitate a clay work session with a group of patients at a cancer outpatient department. The regular group facilitator gave assurances that the group members had shared losses and supported each other through grief and hardship over a period of time. What the author failed to take into account was that she represented an unfamiliar person who was bringing an unknown element into their established group. The group members had no reason to trust the author or the process. As a result, group members kept barriers up as they played with the clay. They produced worms, bowls, the odd flower, and an occasional rude joke. They certainly did not have a cathartic experience or the opportunity to express uncomfortable emotions such as fear, sadness, or anger. Expressing such feelings in the group may have eventuated when they were with each other, but not with a stranger bringing the crazy idea that they should express themselves through clay into their midst.

Another factor that may have been an issue in this group was that they were dealing with current threats. When using clay work to address, for example abuse issues, women are usually dealing with abuse from childhood, past rapes or sexual assaults, or domestic abuse from a previous partner. It is important to feel safe to go home after therapy or a group session. To step out from an intense emotional experience with supportive others into an unsafe environment can leave the client or group member feeling extremely vulnerable. It is always important to ensure that there is safety at home before embarking on clay work. Establishing that clients and group participants have a safe space of their own, and at least one trusted other that they can contact to debrief about residual feelings is essential.

Tips for Practitioners

1. **Large blocks of clay can be bought from pottery or ceramic suppliers, but be careful of your back when lifting and carrying the unprocessed clay; it is heavy.** Terracotta school clay, which has a substantial amount of grit added so that it holds shape, is most suitable.

Terracotta is also good because it is reminiscent of mud and simultaneously has a warm colour. Porcelain or other stoneware has a cold appearance. You will need enough clay so that each participant has a block of at least one-pound weight. A large knife or cheese wire is needed to cut the block of clay into portions. Unused clay can be kept for reuse if it is stored in a sealed plastic bag or bucket with a tight fitting lid.

2. **There is no need for sophisticated tools**. Blunt knives, forks, shaped sticks, chop sticks, and wooden skewers can be useful for shaping and creating surface textures, but the maker's hands are the best tools.

3. **Ban rubber gloves!** Sometimes group participants who are uncomfortable with getting their hands dirty will bring a pair of kitchen gloves; however, the efficacy of clay lies in being in touch with the material. Usually, with humour, it is possible to cajole a participant to try without the gloves. Even reluctant participants find that, despite their initial misgivings, being in touch with clay is pleasurable. Further, emancipation from gloves can be a small act of achievement for someone who is constrained by the need to be constantly clean.

4. **Before beginning, participants need to know that clay has limitations**. It is solid, but wet and will not hold shape if stretched too high or too thin. Such limitations can be useful as metaphors. It is also important to let participants know their models will probably not endure. For clay to be fired it needs to be uniform in thickness and have no air bubbles. Constricting participants to taking the care needed for a firing can limit creativity and spontaneity. Unfired models can be taken home, allowed to dry, and varnished to preserve them if wanted; however, they will be fragile. Often clients and group members take a lump of unmoulded clay home in a plastic bag instead. They can then do further work in their own time.

5. **It is important to free clients and group participants of artistic nerves**. The fear of "not being arty" can be overcome by asking participants to make abstract representations. That means that whatever is produced does not need to look like "something."

6. **Ask participants not to think about what they are making but to let their hands guide them.** Participants may want to sculpt the human form, but this can be frustrating. It may be advisable to ask clients/participants to work in the abstract, which will free people from wrestling with the need to represent the body and end up judging their work as unsatisfactory. Some participants will find this hard and still want to make representations of figures and animals. This is a participant's choice and is not problematic. Some will digress from their objective thought along the way and create something much more valuable from their own mind's eye. This could be because it is much more emancipating to create an imaginative representation of an experience, thought, or feeling that is not constricted by preconceived forms.

7. **Balance difficult emotions with positive feelings**. If a session has focused on traumatic or negative memories, before finishing, ask clients/participants to create a clay model that represents something

positive. This may be their vision for the future, a pleasure in their life now, or something they will do to look after themselves. By doing this, the session ends with feelings of empowerment and hope.

8. **Focus on clients and individual group participants completed clay model.** Ask about what they have created, but it is important that you do not interpret the clay model for them. Your interpretation may be off the mark, and the maker can feel alienated rather than understood

9. **Dry clay is a clean material.** Residual smears dry to a powder that can be brushed from clothing and vacuumed from carpets. However, when wet, clay is exceedingly messy so buckets of water and multiple clean rags are needed for cleanup of worktables. Willing group members who offer to stay back to help with clean up are always valuable. Often during this time, further insights about the experience of clay working are expressed and provide productive insights about process for participants and group facilitators.

10. **Always provide liquid soap and hand cream**. Clay dries the skin, and it is preferable if participants leave with their hands feeling soft and nurtured.

Recommended Readings and Resources

Clay Transformations. (2013). *An innovative research project transforming lives through mural recovery.* Available at: http://www.claytransformations.info/.

Bar-On, T. (2007). A meeting with clay: Individual narratives, self reflection, and action. *Psychology of Aesthetics, Creativity and the Arts, 1*, 225-236.

Malchiodi, C. A. (Ed.). (2011). *Handbook of art therapy.* New York: Guilford Press.

Moon, C. H. (2010). *Materials and media in art therapy.* New York: Routledge.

Sherwood, P. (2004). *The healing art of clay therapy.* Camberwell, Victoria: ACER.

Waldman, J. (1999). Breaking the mould: A woman's psychosocial and artistic journey with clay. *International Journal of Art Therapy: Inscape, 4*(1), 10-19.

References

Anderson, F. E. (1995). Catharsis and empowerment through group claywork with incest survivors. *The Arts in Psychotherapy, 22*(5), 413-427.

Bar-On, T. (2007). A meeting with clay: Individual narratives, self reflection, and action. *Psychology of Aesthetics, Creativity and the Arts, 1*, 225-236

Buchanan, F., Power, C. & Verity, F. (2013). Domestic violence and the place of fear in mother/baby relationships: "What was I afraid of? Of making it worse." *Journal of Interpersonal Violence.* Published online first at http://jiv.sagepub.com/content/early/2013/01/03/0886260512469108. doi: 10.1177/0886260512469108.

Carozza, P. M., & Heirsteiner, C. L. (1982). Young female incest victims in treatment: Stages of growth seen with a group art therapy model. *Clinical Social Work Journal, 10*(3), 165-180.

Dickson-Swift, V., James, E. L., Kippen, S., & Liamputtong, P. (2009). Researching sensitive topics: Qualitative research as emotional work. *Qualitative Research, 9*, 61-79.

Elki-Abuhoff, D. L., Goldblatt, R. B., Gaydos, M., & Corrato, S. (2011). Effects of clay manipulation on somatic dysfunction and emotional distress in patients with Parkinson's disease. *Art Therapy: Journal of the American Art Therapy Association, 25*(3) 122-128.

Friere, P. (1970). *Pedagogy of the oppressed.* New York: Herder & Herder.

Golub, D. (2005). Social action art therapy. *Art Therapy: Journal of the American Art Therapy Association, 22*(1), 17-23.

Henley, D. R. (2002). Facilitating the development of object relations through the use of clay in art therapy. *American Journal of Art Therapy, 29*(3), 69-77.

Herman, J. L. (1992). *Trauma and recovery.* London: Pandora.

Huss, E. (2007). Houses, swimming pools, and thin blonde women: Arts-based research through a critical lens with impoverished Bedouin women. *Qualitative Inquiry, 13*, 960-988.

Kimport, E. R., & Robbins, S. J. (2012). Efficacy of creative clay work for reducing negative mood: A randomized controlled trial. *Art Therapy, 29*(2), 74-79.

McNiff, S. (2011). Artistic expressions as primary modes of inquiry. *British Journal of Guidance & Counselling, 39*, 385-396.

Simons, H., & McCormack, B. (2007). Integrating arts-based inquiry in evaluation methodology: Opportunities and challenges. *Qualitative Inquiry, 13*, 292-311.

Sholt, M., & Gavron, T. (2006). Therapeutic qualities of clay-work in art therapy and psychotherapy: A review. *Art Therapy, 23*(2), 66-72.

Snir, S., & Regev, D. (2012). A dialog with five art materials: Creators share their art making experiences. *The Arts in Psychotherapy, 40*, 94-100

Stuckey, H. L., & Nobel, J. (2010). The connection between art, healing, and public health: A review of current literature. *American Journal of Public Health, 100*(2), 254-264.

Talwar, S. (2007). Accessing traumatic memory through art making: An art therapy protocol. *The Arts in Psychotherapy, 34*, 22-35.

Waller, C. S. (1992). Art therapy with adult incest survivors. *Art Therapy, 9*, 136-138.

Waller, D. (2006) Art therapy for children: How it leads to change. *Clinical Psychology and Psychiatry, 11*(2), 271-282.

Walsh, S. (2006). An Irigarayan framework and resymbolization in an arts-informed research process. *Qualitative Inquiry, 12*, 976-993.

Chapter 7: Realities, Facts, and Fiction: Lessons Learned through Storytelling

Jill M. Chonody & Donna Wang

Introduction

Storytelling is a powerful age-old art form. It is a method of self-expression, a way to connect with others, and one of the few universal things shared by people across age, race, culture, and religion. Humans are natural storytellers, and it appears to be a fundamental way that we express ourselves. As young children we are told or read stories, and beginning at an early age, we tell our own stories. Whether we are trying to explain something to another person or engaging in everyday conversations, most of the time, we are telling a story. Oftentimes, these stories are used to communicate meaning to another person rather than to merely relay factual information (McAdams, 1993).

Recollecting stories often provokes nostalgia for a time, place, or person. Its power sheds wisdom throughout the ages and passes down knowledge, information, and history between generations, preserving collective history and culture. Stories are also passed down by family members, which collectively create the history and culture for that family. When these stories are told and re-told, they become a "family story" and important information is communicated about the family system. The re-telling of these stories helps to strengthen the bonds between family members and propels the personal history of the family through these stories (Atkinson, 1995). This type of storytelling may be used as an approach to practice and is found in several models of therapy, such as life review and reminiscence therapy, which is commonly used with older adults or narrative therapy, which seeks to help clients re-author their personal narratives to highlight hope, strengths, and change. Therapeutic benefits of storytelling include catharsis and empowerment for the person telling the story, and connection and healing for those hearing the story.

Likewise, storytelling is represented in creative forms of expression, including fiction and poetry. Both forms of expression may be used to generate entertainment, but they are also an art form that speaks to larger human truths. Storytelling groups that make use of fictional writing can assist participants in understanding or relating to difficult tasks or ideas and may be used as a way to process life experiences. Poetry can also be a vehicle for self-expression but it does not have to adhere to traditional modes of storytelling and lends well to public presentations, such as a spoken word event.

The purpose of this chapter is to provide an overview of these different types of storytelling methods, and the way each are used to engage and benefit individuals, groups, and community. Storytelling groups and activities can provide both a creative outlet and lead to personal change. Relevant literature on effectiveness as well as tips and examples are presented for groups that commonly use storytelling as a therapeutic method.

Life Review and Reminiscence

Life review and reminiscence therapy are techniques that seek to provide a process for "thinking and talking about one's life" (Buchannan et al. 2002, p. 134). Individuals recall past experiences and are then encouraged to share them out loud, often in the form of a story. Both approaches are commonly used with older adults, and this recollection/review is believed to be a necessary task as one comes to the realization that her/his life is coming to an end (Butler, 1963). Therefore, older adults may feel a need to integrate their life experiences and tie up "loose ends" (Soltys & Kunz, 2007). As a result, they may experience a new perspective, closure, gratification, and/or resolution (Soltys & Kunz, 2007).

Life review is a structured method, which includes a critical examination of past experiences throughout the entire life span (Buchannan et al., 2002). Each time period (e.g., childhood) is reviewed in full before moving to the next period. This process of review is therapeutic in nature, and the goal is to achieve a resolution of earlier issues, which allows the individual to feel at ease with the past (Richeson & Thorson, 2002). For example, a person may be asked to recall a difficult situation in her/his life and to discuss how s/he coped with it. From a therapeutic standpoint, this may help the individual identify strengths or skills that can be used in a present situation or to learn from those past mistakes and approach a similar problem differently. This technique requires participants to have advanced introspection skills (Coleman, 2005), and because groups are therapeutic in nature, a practitioner or someone with training in therapeutic groups needs to lead or co-lead the activity.

On the other hand, reminiscence is an unstructured version of the life review process whereby the individual decides what stories to share. Reminiscence is not guided by the underlying goal that conflict from the past necessarily needs to achieve a resolution (Jones & Beck-Little, 2002). In that way, it is less specifically therapeutic in its goals. Rather, this approach seeks to provide a space for storytelling; something that all of us are compelled to do. It typically occurs in a group setting, and the process of sharing personal stories may facilitate new relationships (Coleman, 2005) and reduce social isolation (Buchannan et al., 2002).

Regardless of the approach used, research indicates that capacity for growth and ability to creatively express oneself continues to occur regardless of age (Cohen, 2001, 2006). In other words, storytelling and other creative activities are useful techniques that can lead to positive changes when working with older adults, even for those who are experiencing cognitive impairment (e.g., dementia). Results from multiple studies suggest that older people with cognitive decline benefit from reminiscence activities, including a decrease in agitation (Hagens, Beaman, & Ryan, 2003), increased well-being (Lai, Chi, & Kayser-Jones, 2004), and improved life satisfaction (Bohlmeijer, Smit, & Cuijpers 2007). Furthermore, reminiscence can help reduce depression, increase life satisfaction, improve self-care and self-esteem, and help older adults deal with crises, losses, and transitions (Jones & Beck-Little, 2002). Better outcomes for nursing home residents have also been found, including a positive impact on emotional well-being and cognitive functioning (see Parker, 1995 and Buchanan et al., 2002 for a review of outcomes).

Storytelling through reminiscence or life review offers a straightforward technique for engagement with groups, and as such, would lend well to combining various mediums to promote group goals. Other techniques may include an exploration of mementos, photographs, journals, or other memorabilia, which in turn, could facilitate greater resolution or further exploration of past experiences (Zalaquett & Stens, 2006) or could simply be used to create group cohesion and facilitate the process of participants getting to know one another. For example, Hagens et al. (2003) combine reminiscence activities for cognitively impaired residents of a long-term care facility, which were utilized to create "Remembering Boxes." These boxes contained writings and meaningful personal objects. In addition to a reduction in agitation for residents, these boxes also facilitated conversation between residents and staff and improved interactions between residents and their family. Regardless of the group goals, storytelling and reminiscence can be used to enhance those efforts, either through a one-time activity or the incorporation of storytelling throughout the group process.

While life review and reminiscence are typically used with older adults, there is no reason that these processes could not be used with other individuals, including youth. For some young people, a lot of experiences have occurred in their short lives, and the way these experiences might be integrated and re-processed could be beneficial. The life review process may be most useful for achieving therapeutic goals, but reminiscence may be a better approach across the life span given that it is not intended for one specific reason. For example, middle school or high school youth may use a reminiscence type program to build relationships through group process and develop additional social skills. Given that "reminiscence is a reflexive process," individuals can "introspectively define (or redefine) themselves" at any age (Parker, 1995, p. 515). The process of talking with another person about the past creates the context for greater understanding of the self. "The principal method by which individuals validate their existence is through speech" (Parker, 1995, p. 516), and as such, reminiscence groups can provide that opportunity to talk through both the past and the present by storytelling.

Another alternative to personal reminiscence may be the life story interview. Atkinson (1995) indicates, "an experience equally powerful to writing your own autobiography…is interviewing someone else for their life story" (p. 115). This approach could be used to create or strengthen intergenerational relationships by having young people interview their grandparents or other older adults in their life. It may also be useful for adults to interview one another and gather the other person's life history. Writings could be created or the activity could be used to generate interpersonal relationships, social skill development, or enhanced communication. In sum, the process of storytelling and reminiscing offer a wide range of possibilities for working with groups and individuals.

Case example: Incorporating Technology, Social Media, and Group Process into Storytelling

"The Best Day of My Life So Far" is a storytelling group for older adults at a senior center in Philadelphia, but it is also much more. The group began as the result of a very personal experience for the founder, Benita Cooper. Benita began having a conversation with her grandmother—the first real dialogue that she had ever had with her and they haven't stopped talking since (read the full story here: http://www.fooklingbenitacooper.com/). In 2009, Benita decided to take this experience to the community and began a group with older adults at the Philadelphia Senior Center, which was originally supposed to last for 6 weeks—it is still going (a documentary video is available online that describes the class and introduces the seniors; view it here: www.youtube.com/watch?v=l3ZAb8o0 FAg&feature=c4-overview-vl&list=PLAF08A55BC9CD7984).

The class meets once a week for about an hour and is part storytelling group and part "party time" as the members describe it. The class is open to anyone and attendance varies slightly from week to week with a core of members who have been attending since it first began. At the beginning of class, seniors are given about ten minutes to write a story, which might be about a recent event or a distant memory. After the writing time is complete, each person takes a turn reading their story to the group. These stories then form the basis of a blog (view it here: http://blog.bestdayofmylifesofar.org/), which is supplemented with pictures, media, fundraising activities, and posts by Benita. The blog is intended to honor the stories, poems, and sometimes drawings that members create during class, and it also serves as a bridge for friends, family, and the general public to read about the lives of older adults. Moreover, this program seeks to connect people across generations (Chonody & Wang, 2013), as intergenerational activities have been shown to improve younger people's attitudes towards older people and vice-a-versa (Wenzel & Rensen, 2000).

Utilizing multiple forms of technology, this program seeks to empower older adults to reach their full potential and embrace new life experiences. The storytelling aspect of the project is just one of the ways that this program is beneficial to members. A significant social component takes places as stories are shared. People get to know one another through these stories and have the opportunity to laugh, learn, and grieve right alongside the storyteller. When seniors come week after week, the group becomes a new source of friendship where they slowly get to know one another through this sharing activity. Some members even spend time outside the class—drinking coffee, seeing movies, or attending a Chinese New Year celebration. Each of these aspects of the group may be transformative for a member who may have to come the group socially isolated, lonely, or depressed.

This program represents a blend of an older technique with a new spin. Past research supports the benefits of storytelling and reminiscence for older adults

(Bohlmeijer et al., 2003), but "The Best Day of My Life So Far" brings that into the new technological age with a blog, a Facebook page, twitter account, and Youtube videos (see: http://www.youtube.com/user/bestdaysofar). Innovative program development may facilitate increased intergenerational connection and renewed communication amongst family members in addition to giving older adults a forum to share stories and build new relationships. This one storytelling group is also on its way to expanding into a national network of many more groups with connected blogs, which may help further bridge communication, relationships, and mutual sharing.

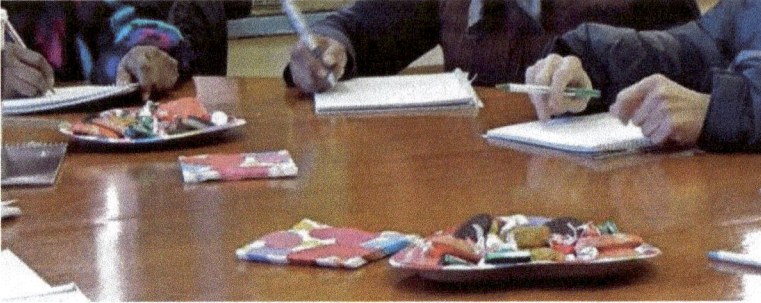

Title: Storytelling Group.
Location: Philadelphia, PA.
Photo by: Jill Chonody.

The Nuns 12/22/09

Aunt Nancy had taught me to read before I was four years old. After my fifth birthday in June 1949 she asked me if I would like to go to first grade in September or wait another year. Fortunately, I chose to wait and I was still the shortest and lightest boy in my grade all through the eight years of elementary school. When my mother introduced me to the wonderful principal the first day I couldn't wait to get home and

ask "Mom why the "Sisters" all dressed like witches.

Title: The Nuns.
Story by: Mo McCooper.

Narrative Therapy

The underpinning of narrative therapy is the belief that reality is determined by social perspective and interaction. Multiple stories thus create our shared reality, and no one narrative is more "true" than another. The events of our life, even day-to-day life, are linked together through the interpretation and meaning that are assigned to these events, and a story is created from this interplay. Everyone is living a multi-storied life, and no single story fully encompasses all aspects of the event. Moreover, multiple stories may be told about the same occurrence with each teller emphasizing or privileging certain facets of the event, which fit into the overall story. It is through sharing of personal narratives that we determine and solidify our identities, and life stories illustrate who we are and how we feel about our life, our future, ourselves, and our relationships. Thus, a client's stories play a key role in narrative therapy, and as such, represent the essence of the work that is to occur during the therapeutic process (Morgan, 2000). In other words, storytelling provides the vehicle for creating identity and is purposefully used in narrative therapy as a healing mechanism.

In narrative therapy, clients seek to change their narrative and thus reformulate their identity. The goal of the therapeutic process is to "re-story" conversations and events. The practitioner helps the client seek out other meanings to their stories and to find alternative stories that s/he would like to live (Morgan, 2000). Moreover, the meaning that is attributed to individual stories is challenged to help the client recreate the stories. Narrative therapy has been found to be useful in a number of studies, including parent/child conflicts (Besa, 1994), post-traumatic stress in refugees (Neuner, Schauer, Klaschik, Karunakara, & Elbert, 2004), and adults with major depressive disorder (Vromans & Schweitzer, 2011). Etchison and Kleist (2000) indicate that narrative therapy is also beneficial in the context of family therapy and may be applicable across a range of issues.

Additional training in the techniques of narrative therapy is essential to good practice of this approach; however, clinicians are likely already aware that most therapy sessions incorporate storytelling, and the meaning behind these stories may become a focus of intervention. Resources regarding narrative therapy are available online from the Dulwich Centre (see *Recommended Readings and Resources*) and numerous books and in-person training opportunities are available.

Creative Storytelling: Fiction and Poetry

Fiction and poetry can be thought of as an "empty basket," just waiting to be filled with whatever a person chooses. It can be filled with sweet fruit, dried twigs, or building blocks. One of the key things is: it is up to the writer. The journey or story that that the writer would like to tell, the meaning, and the intended impact will all drive the structure of the writing. Although a dearth of research exists regarding the application and outcomes of fiction and poetry in practice, the potential for personal growth and empowerment is difficult to deny. Both approaches are explored here within the context of working with individuals and groups to achieve personal enrichment and create meaning.

Fiction

Fictional writing is always based in a kind of reality, that of the fundamental human experience. Seven basic plots serve as the foundation for all stories: 1) person vs. nature; 2) person vs. person; 3) person vs. the environment; 4) person vs. machines/technology; 5) person vs. the supernatural; 6) person vs. self; and 7) person vs. god/religion. The essence or the meaning of stories that are told will involve one or more of these central themes, and such, this supports the power of storytelling to reach those universal truths of the human experience. Each of these elements are known to us at an essential level and contribute to our desire to read or view the "stories" that are played out through popular mediums, such as movies and books. Furthermore, every one of us has a story—our story, which can be converted into other forms, and have the potential to "take us even closer to experiences than verbatim descriptions" (McNiff, 2007, p. 38)

Fictional writing is likely to be only thinly veiled autobiographical information (Murray, 1991), and at the very least, most writers draw from their own experiences to create their stories. Therefore, using these stories as a springboard, individuals can transform their experiences into short stories, novels, or other forms of fictional writing as a way to achieve healing, humor, or to connect with others. The shared human experience that is illustrated in fictional works makes this type of storytelling and writing a potentially powerful approach to working with various groups. "Fictional explorations allows us penetrate more freely and intimately into the particular subject matter, to identify with the characters and situations in new ways, and to speak from the perspectives of others" (McNiff, 2007, p. 38). For example, people who have experienced trauma may tap into their journey of recovery to create a fictional story that illustrates hope and perseverance. For some, the veil of anonymity that is created by fictionalizing personal information may provide a freedom to open up about difficult thoughts, feelings, and experiences. While this approach does not have a research base per se, therapeutic writing has been shown to be physically and psychologically beneficial (Wright & Chung, 2001). For example, patients with chronic illness were shown to have significant improvements when they wrote about their stressful life experiences (Smyth, Stone, Hurewitz, & Kabell, 1999). Translating that to fictional writing is a logical next step and may provide an alternative method to traditional journaling and storytelling.

Poetry

> Poetry is just the evidence of life. If your life is burning well, poetry is just the ash. ~ Leonard Cohen

Poetry provides the opportunity to delve deeply into one's most private and intimate experiences, which are "distilled, pared to succinctness, and made music to the ear by lyricism" (Bolton, 1999, p. 118). It is a "snippet of human experience that is artistically expressed" (Leavy, 2009, p. 64). The use of poetry and poetry writing may be implemented with different groups to achieve a variety of goals, including therapeutic objectives. In this context, poetry writing provides a catharsis for the writer and a technique for exploring thoughts, feelings, and experiences. Writing poetry is a form of therapeutic writing, and a pilot project in the United Kingdom suggests that this type of writing was beneficial for those patients who were experiencing problems in their life (Bolton, 1998).

In poetry writing, both product and process are essential to change. Bolton (1999) states, "In the ten years I have been working in therapeutic writing, I have never known anyone to write anything which is not the right thing—painful and distressing to deal with perhaps—but always right for that writer at that time" (p. 121). In terms of process, the re-writing or re-working of those initial thoughts and feelings can bring new insight (Bolton, 1999). The product is that final representation of the change process, which creates context and meaning for life experiences. Creating a poem goes through this evolution of change—initializing the writing, changing it, re-writing it, and then finalizing its form. This process and the eventual product not only represent the changes in the person, but also that process of achieving it.

Furthermore, the use of poetry writing as a therapeutic technique may be especially appropriate during particular life stages. Preliminary findings indicate that writing poetry may be helpful for those who are facing end-of-life issues (Bolton, 1999). Much like the process of reminiscence or life review, people who are dying may have a need to express themselves and understand past issues. Thus, writing poetry may provide an alternative approach to life review or be used as adjunct to that process. Similarly, poetry may also be useful people who are experiencing depression or anxiety. Client changes, both physiologically and psychologically, have been documented as the result of therapeutic writing (e.g., Pennebaker, 1989).

The inclusion of performance with poetry writing may also be advantageous when working with groups, particularly youth. Bruce and Davis (2000) discuss how the use of poetry may be useful in preventing violence amongst adolescents whereby youth are helped to "find words that will in turn help them to identify, clarify, express, and channel thoughts and feelings rather than act either inwardly or outwardly violent" (p. 121). In this innovative approach, a "hip-hop pedagogy" was utilized as an alternative approach to work with students, which allowed teachers to connect with students in a realm of poetry that they already knew. To support their overall curriculum of "Nonviolence and Leadership Poetry Workshops," a poetry slam was planned. This allows people access to poetry— even for those who feel like poetry is "impenetrable" (Bruce & Davis, 2000). This public presentation of poetry provides an outlet for the thoughts, feelings, ideas, and words that are already present inside each person with the goal of "show[ing] students the power of words in order to instruct them in nonviolence, leadership, character, and social change" (Bruce & Davis, 2000, p. 124). When working with youth, an approach such as this could provide the ideal context for exploring larger issues within their lives and the community. By starting with a knowledge base that is shared amongst adolescents, the move toward personal change or empowerment may be facilitated with ease.

In sum, the diversity of reasons to write poetry is best illustrated when writer Sage Cohen (2009) asked five women, "why do you write poetry?" They responded:

To bear witness;

> Because in writing, I can be anyone;
> To stay engaged with my own divinity;
> Unlike life, nothing is permanent in writing—everything is malleable;
> To change the world (p. 3).

These responses exemplify the wealth of diversity in what poetry writing can mean to the writer. This creative outlet provides the freedom to tell one's story or point of view without the constraints of traditional approaches to storytelling that are primarily driven by plot. Moreover, written poetry can then be performed to create an experience for the listener as well as the performer. Poetry slams and spoken word performances are becoming increasingly more popular and can be powerful tribute to life experiences and human emotion.

The Use of Stories to Build and Strengthen Community

In the most simple of logic, storytelling creates community by connecting two individuals—the storyteller and the listener; however, cultivating community obviously goes far deeper and is achieved via different routes. One way that community is generated via storytelling is the preservation of culture. Vanessa Jackson (undated) writes,

> The telling of stories has been an integral part of the history of people of African descent. From the Griots of ancient African to the sometimes painful lyrics of hip-hop artists, people of African descent have known that our lives and our stories must be spoken, over and over again, so that the people will know our truth (p. 2).

Although certain aspects of life will likely go formally undocumented, perhaps the best way to preserve information is through storytelling or "oral tradition." Personal and family stories are preserved this way but a community can also be maintained in a similar way. Community can be generated via similar interests whereby people come together with a common goal. Coskie, Trudel, and Vohs (2010) describe how storytelling was used to help a class of third-graders come out of their shell, build skills, and connect with one another. In instances like these, stories are an avenue to develop the skills and ability to work in a group or a community and to further enhance oneself. Similarly, Schuster (1998) reports that the creation of a writing group in a long-term nursing facility helped participants form their own community within the larger community. This creation of community in turn propelled a change in these residents in terms of their sense of self and their relationships with other people. These studies illustrate how a community can be created and transformed through writing and storytelling.

With ever-changing technology, community does not have to have walls, and virtual communities are ever increasing. Repositories of stories, such as cowbird.com, are innovative ways to create community through modern technology. For example, a photojournalist who was struggling to capture the true essence of a Native American reservation received help when members of the reservation began flooding him with stories, song, and pictures to tell their stories, and how they live their lives (see http://ngm.nationalgeographic.com/2012/08/pine-ridge/community-project-intro). People with similar interests, or stories, now have a way to connect without even meeting face-to-face.

Storytelling can also be used to create change within the broader community. One approach to this is through the use of narrative therapy principles. For example, in response to requests from community members with mental health issues, a strengths-based, community approach was implemented by therapists to help these individuals with daily tasks (Freedman & Combs, 2009). Community support workers along with the therapists implemented a program that offered community-based assistance in an effort to skirt outcomes associated with pathology-based approaches to treating mental health (i.e., psychiatric hospitalization), which can leave people feeling demoralized (Freedman & Combs, 2009). Thus, a new narrative can be created regarding mental health and treatment for those who are struggling.

Another narrative based approach is community gatherings. These events have been held across Australia at the request of different groups, including people experiencing mental illness, people living with HIV (Denborough, 2002), and Aboriginal Australians who wish to address suicide prevention on the lands (Denborough et al., 2006). An essential component of narrative therapy is to understand the knowledge and skills present in the community and to document the ways in which these resources can be used to solve current issues (Denborough, 2002). At these gatherings, conversations regarding their resources are facilitated and recorded. Discussing and sharing ideas about these resources out loud in a public forum is a way of reinforcing the presence of positive community assets. Gatherings also typically include a collection of stories, songs, and ideas, and as the process unfolds, community members guide and shape the gathering, not the facilitators. Members retain ownership of the recordings that are created, which can then be used for future re-tellings of the stories and community sharing (Denborough et al., 2006).

Furthermore, cultural narratives can be altered through the process of storytelling. Some narratives act to devalue a certain group of people, which can in turn be incorporated into personal narratives (Rappaport, 1995). However, these narratives can be challenged, leading to empowerment and increased awareness in the community. For example, social narratives may propel the belief that most gay men are HIV+. Gay men may seek to work together to change this narrative. With collective effort, their stories of prejudice and oppression could be shared within the community to illustrate how these beliefs are harmful. This approach may also be used for educational purposes. For example, Salzer (1998) used this approach to examine the writings of college students about public housing to explore how social discourse on poverty influenced student perceptions. Applying this method to other groups, change may be elicited both within the group as well as in the broader community context. For example, when working with a group of youth, they could be asked to write narratives about their community. Their essays could then be examined and explored with the goal of understanding how dominant social narratives influence personal narratives. These explorations may then be used to create community projects that seek to delve deeper into the issues that were raised within the group. In sum, storytelling is an essential component of a community and is a process that can be used create, maintain, or change a community.

Benefits and Potential Challenges

The use of storytelling has many benefits to the practitioner as well as to the individual whose story is shared. For the practitioner, benefits include that it is low to no cost, and it does not require special space or equipment. Verbal storytelling also does not require a level of literacy, making it accessible for those who might have limited reading or writing skills or individuals of varying cognitive functioning (Zalaquett & Stens, 2006).

Another benefit is its versatility. Storytelling is useful one-on-one or in a group and can be modified in different ways (e.g., an object can be brought into the session and stories could be written about it or what it makes you think about). Storytelling can also be used in conjunction with other creative endeavors (e.g., photography, painting, drawing) and use multiple methods for communication. For example, aside from the obvious verbal storytelling, stories can be told through art, dance, or wikis. This may also provide an opportunity for a person to either communicate in a way that s/he is comfortable or perhaps try a new creative outlet.

Storytelling can also be a way to connect different generations and cultures, while celebrating and honoring differences. There have been instances where when someone hears of a story from another culture, that person recognizes a similar story or moral from their culture. Decreasing the divide, improving awareness and/or increasing one's understanding of various cultures may bridge similarities. As it has been suggested throughout the humanities, "there is more that binds us as human beings than there are differences." The point is, we are all human and carry the human experience of emotions, challenges, and happiness, regardless of race, ethnicity, age, sex, sexual orientation, ability, or religion.

One potential challenge to consider when in a group setting is language abilities. Issues such as not speaking the primary language as well as levels of functioning may interfere with an individual's ability to fully participate. For example, some older adults lose capacity to speak at loud volumes, thus not being able to hear them could be an issue and lead to disinterest by the listeners. Other activities that facilitate storytelling may be beneficial, such as one-on-one interactions or non-vocal storytelling. Alternatively, it is possible to incorporate the strengths of other group members to help or "mentor" others that may have special challenges or issues.

Without a doubt, some stories are hard to hear. The listener needs to be aware of what "buttons" are being pushed or perhaps bringing up personal issues. Whatever the case may be, the listener needs to be in tune with the present moment. Overall, it may be helpful to remain focused on the bigger picture. For example, listening for the meaning of the story, rather than focusing on the details of the story may be beneficial. Likewise, when working with older adults through reminiscence activities, the issue of death is likely to arise. Individuals should consider how they have worked through their personal anxiety regarding mortality and their level of comfort with the topic prior to starting the group (Barry, 1988). Moreover, this topic may emerge in various forms across other age ranges, and if parameters around certain topics are warranted, then these should be considered and discussed up front with the group. Practitioners should also be comfortable stopping the discussion if the content is inappropriate (Jones & Beck-Little, 2002).

Understand that for some people and situations, telling a story is taking a risk for them. Within these stories may be personal hurt or shame. A discussion prior to story sharing may include monitoring one's own reactions. For example, listeners may want to laugh during a story when in fact the storyteller is not intending to be funny. Likewise, some stories are very important and meaningful to some people (e.g., stories from religious texts) and should never be treated as casual or insignificant. Inappropriate reactions may be humiliating and hurtful to the storyteller.

Ethical Considerations

One of the key challenges of reminiscence work or other autobiographical driven activities is that intense emotions may be revealed in the storytelling process (Barry, 1988). It may uncover unpleasant thoughts or memories and may stir intense emotions, such as sadness, anger, or anxiety. Sharing stories that may have been repressed can conjure up very intense emotions for the person and remind her/him of the trauma. Thus, when a person tells a story, some re-victimization of the storyteller may occur. While this is a common outcome in therapeutic contexts, if working in a different milieu, then a plan of action should be considered in case this issue should arise. The practitioner needs to be ready to provide appropriate follow-up as needed (Wang, 2011), such as community referrals or additional support in the moment.

If storytelling is done in a group setting, there is also the concern of how the story may evoke strong emotions among the group members. Hence a practitioner should follow the basic guidelines for running therapeutic groups, such as setting ground rules as well as other ethical considerations that exist in more traditional therapeutic relationships. For example, a discussion of confidentiality up front will help in the long run to create a space where all feel safe to share and express their viewpoints and experiences. Practitioners need to be sure that group members are aware that the stories that are told or other information that is revealed (such as trauma or abuse) should be treated as private.

Finally, when working with individuals or groups on fictional writings or poetry, issues related to ownership may arise. The individual should retain the use of their writings, and the writer should determine if or when they are used in other contexts. In some settings, such as nursing homes or community care, creative products that are generated within classes are used for marketing, fundraising, and other community events. Writers should be able to consent to these uses and retain ownership over their work.

Tips for Practitioners

1. **Storytelling efforts may need to take a therapeutic approach if the emotional well-being of group members is of concern.** Thus, they need to be lead or co-lead by someone with training and experience in

group therapy. For example, if planning a storytelling group with adolescents who are known to have experienced past trauma, special care should be taken to plan ahead for possible emotional repercussions in the group.

2. **Storytelling activities can be combined with other creative approaches and new technologies to enhance its effects.** As illustrated in the case example, use of social media and a blog creates additional opportunities for emotional bonding, both within the family and the larger community. Using different modes of technology may enhance the approach or interest in storytelling and may also create additional, tangible benefits, such as learning a new skill. If stories are used in public ways (i.e., online), then the issue of consent should be negotiated upfront. Other combination possibilities could include storytelling and photography. Participants could take pictures to illustrate stories, use photographs of favorite objects to tell stories, or prompts could be used to generate photographs, which in turn, could be used for storytelling. For example, participants could be asked, "What is your life like?" and then asked to take pictures. Upon returning to the group, each participant could choose one of her/his photographs and tell the story. Alternatively, photographs from magazines could be brought into the group, and once participants have chosen a picture, they can take turns creating a story to go with the picture (Chonody, Martin, Amitrani-Welsh, 2014).

3. **To stimulate reminiscence, consider the use of sketching or writing as a first step.** Alternatively, memorabilia, such as old photographs and letters, may stimulate memories about the past. These approaches may be particularly useful when running a reminiscence group for individuals with cognitive impairment. In addition, Barry (1988) suggests the use of an outline, which includes developmental time periods (e.g., early years) and subjects (e.g., school days). These techniques may be used to generate further storytelling and reminiscence with different groups.

4. **When running a storytelling group, setting ground rules with the group may facilitate smooth running of these meetings.** For example, setting a time limit for storytelling may be helpful or necessary when the session is time-limited or for participants who are particularly verbose. A discussion of confidentiality and other ways that stories or poems may be used should also be done upfront, and group members should have the opportunity to opt out of any public sharing that is planned.

5. **The use of metaphors may help participants gain greater understanding of the writing process and the skills needed to achieve their personal goals.** Westcott (1997) makes use of photographic procedures as a metaphor to explore the writing process and its components. For example, all photographs make use of focus to illustrate a certain aspect of a scene. Just like a good photograph, writing needs a specific focus to capture the readers' attention. Sometimes stories contain too many details or facts, and the important parts of the story become lost in the background (Westcott, 1997). Even if the writing skill is not meant to produce professional stories, additional

information and skill building can help participants feel more confident and comfortable with tackling a new creative endeavor.

6. **Storytelling is very versatile and activities may be incorporated into programs designed for children, older adults, or patients in hospital/hospice settings.** When done in a group, stories may be written prior to the session, and the writer can read or paraphrase what has been written. Alternatively, spontaneous storytelling can be utilized as an impromptu activity. For example, ask participants to tell a story about the last time they laughed really hard or to describe their strangest habit.

7. **Consider the use of community gatherings or spoken word events.** This may be a way to promote strengths and showcase resilience amongst a group of people. One such event occurred in Philadelphia amongst participants of the *Best Day of My Life, So Far* whereby older adults shared a story of their choosing in front of an audience. It represented an opportunity to showcase the vitality and humor of old adults and challenge the notion that older people cannot be fun. On the other hand, a poetry reading or spoken word event can be organized to challenge the dominant social discourse. For example, written pieces regarding race and the experiences associated with it could be used as a theme to illustrate diversity within racial/ethnic groups.

8. **Recognize that poetry and fiction can take many forms**. For example, in poetry, rhyming or certain patterns, such as haiku cold be used. Giving participants concrete parameters could be helpful to jumpstart a project, but allowing participants to blur lines can also provide for a freedom of expression. Be open to either or to using multiple approaches!

9. **Try incorporating other storytelling methods from time to time.** Whether running a traditional storytelling group, regardless if it is reminiscence-based or fiction, variety may be a way to enhance the primary goals of the group. For example, the life story interview may provide a new opportunity for fictional writers to explore the perspective of another person. By sharing this interview with the group, fictional stories may be generated.

10. **Regardless if the stories are fact or fiction, create a book with group participants**. *Blurb* offers free software that creates a layout for the written text and provides plenty of space for photographs or other items. While printing costs could be problematic, smaller, paperback versions can be generated through the software and would be a nice memento of the group experience, particularly if the program is time-limited.

Recommended Readings and Resources

Atkinson, R. (1995). *The gift of stories: Practical and spiritual applications of autobiography, life stories, and personal mythmaking*. Westport, CT: Bergin & Garvey.

Biren, J. E., & Deutchman, D. E. (1991). *Guiding autobiography groups for older adults: Exploring the fabric of life*. Baltimore, MA: John Hopkins.

Blanch, A., Filson, B., & Penney, D. (2012). Trauma-informed storytelling and other healing practices. In *Engaging women in trauma-informed peer support: A guidebook* (Chapter 11). Available at: www.ct.gov/dmhas/lib/dmhas/trauma/EngagingWomen.pdf.

Blurb. (2013). *Create your own book.* Available at: http://www.blurb.com/.

Community Expressions. (2013). *Enhancing community connections through storytelling.* Available at: http://digitalexploration.org/resources/storytelling/.

Dulwich Centre. (2013). *Dulwich Centre: A gateway to narrative therapy and community work.* Resources on narrative therapy available at: www.dulwichcentre.com.au/.

Haugh, E. K., Murray, S., Elle, J., Bach, J., Basden, R., Chisolm, S., Crow, D., Easterling, V. J., Federenko, E., Gorey, M., Longway, T., Matthews, R., & Trammell, J. (2002). Teacher to teacher: What is your favourite activity for teaching poetry. *Teaching and Writing Poetry, 91*(3), 2-31.

Mazza, N. F. (2003). *Poetry therapy: Theory and practice.* New York: Routledge.

Struthers, R. (2006). Storytelling. In M. Snyder & R. Lindquist (Eds.), *Complementary and alternative therapies in nursing* (5th ed., pp. 153-164). New York: Springer.

Transom. (2013). *A showcase & workshop for new public radio.* Resources for recording stories available at: http://transom.org/.

References

Atkinson, R. (1995). *The gift of stories: Practical and spiritual applications of autobiography, life stories, and personal mythmaking.* Westport, CT: Bergin & Garvey.

Barry, J. (1988). Autobiographical writing: An effective tool for practice with the oldest old. *Social work, 33*(5), 449-451.

Besa, D. (1994). Evaluating narrative family therapy using single-system research designs. *Research on Social Work Practice, 4*(3), 309-325.

Bohlmeijer, E., Smit, F., & Cuijpers, P. (2003). Effects of reminiscence and life review on late-life depression: A meta-analysis. *International Journal of Geriatric Psychiatry, 18*, 1088-1094.

Bolton, G. (1999). Every poem breaks a silence that had to be overcome: The therapeutic power of poetry writing. *Feminist Review, 62*, 118-133.

Bolton, G. (1998). Writing not pills: Writing therapy in primary care. In C. Hunt & F. Samson (Eds.), *The self on the page: Theory and practice of creative writing in personal development* (pp. 78-92). London: Jessica Kingsley.

Bruce, H. E., & Davis, B. D. (2000). Slam: Hip-hop meets poetry—A strategy for violence intervention. *The English Journal, 89*(5), 119-127.

Buchanan, D., Moorhouse, A., Cabico, L., Krock, M., Campbell, H., & Spevakow, D. (2002). A critical review and synthesis of literature on reminiscing with older adults. *Canadian Journal of Nursing Research, 34*(3), 123-139.

Butler, R. N. (1963). The life review: An interpretation of reminiscence in the aged. *Psychiatry, 26*, 486-496.

Chonody, J. M., Martin, T., & Amitrani-Welsh, J. (2014). Looking through the lens of urban teenagers: Reflections on participatory photography in an alternative high school. *Reflections: Narratives of Professional Helping, 18,* 35-44.

Chonody, J.M., & Wang, D. (2013). Connecting older adults to the community through multimedia: An intergenerational reminiscence program. *Activities, Adaptation, and Aging, 37*(1), 79-93.

Cohen, G. D. (2001). Creativity with aging: Four phases of potential in the second half of life. *Geriatrics, 58*(2), 51-57.

Cohen, G. D. (2006). Research on creativity and aging: The positive impact of the arts on health and illness. *Generations, 30*(1), 7-15.

Cohen, S. (2009). *Writing the life poetic: An invitation to read and write poetry.* Cincinnati, OH: Writer's Digest.

Coleman, P. G. (2005). Reminiscence: Developmental, social and clinical perspectives. In M. L. Johnson (Ed.), *The Cambridge handbook of age and ageing* (pp. 301-309). Cambridge: Cambridge University Press.

Coskie, T., Trudel, H., & Vohs, R. (2010). Creating community through storytelling. *Talking Points, 22*(1), 2-9.

Denborough, D. (2002). Community song writing and narrative practice. *Clinical Psychology, 17,* 17-24.

Denborough, D., Koolmatrie, C., Mununggirritj, D., Marika, D., Dhurrkay, W., & Yunupingu, M. (2006). Linking stories and initiatives: A narrative approach to working with the skills and knowledge of communities. *The International Journal of Narrative Therapy and Community Work, 2,* 19-51.

Etchison, M., & Kleist, D. M. (2000). Review of narrative therapy: Research and utility. *The Family Journal, 8,* 61-66.

Freedman, J., & Combs, G. (2009). Narrative ideas for consulting with communities and organizations: Ripples from the gatherings. *Family Process, 48*(3), 347-362.

Hagens, C., Beaman, A., & Ryan, E. B. (2003). Reminiscing, poetry writing, and remembering boxes: Personhood-centered communication with cognitively impaired adults. *Activities, Adaptation, & Aging, 27(3/4),* 97-112.

Jackson, V. (undated). *In our own voice: African-American stories of oppression, survival and recovery in the mental health system.* Retrieved from www.healingcircles.org/uploads/INOVweb.pdf.

Jones, E., & Beck-Little, R. (2002). The use of reminiscence therapy for the treatment of depression in rural-dwelling older adults. *Issues in Mental Health Nursing, 23*(3), 279-290.

Lai, K. Y., Chi, I., & Kayser-Jones, J. S. (2004). A randomized controlled trial of specific reminiscence approach to promote the well-being of nursing home residents with dementia. *International Psychogeriatrics, 16*(1), 33-49.

Leavy, P. (2009). *Method meets art: Arts-based research practice.* New York: Guilford.

McAdams, D. P. (1993). The meaning of stories. In *Stories we live by: Personal myths and the making of the self* (pp. 19-37). New York: Guildford.

McNiff, S. (2007). Art-based research. In J. Gary & A. L. Cole (Eds.), *Handbook of arts in qualitative research: Perspectives, methodologies, examples, and issues* (pp. 29-40). Thousand Oaks, CA: Sage.

Morgan, A. (2000). *What is narrative therapy? An easy to read introduction.* Adelaide, South Australia: Dulwich Centre Publications.

Murray, D. M. (1991). All writing is autobiography. *College Composition and Communication, 42*(1), 66-74.

Neuner, F., Schauer, M., Klaschik, C., Karunakara, U., & Elbert, T. (2004). A comparison of narrative exposure therapy, supportive counseling, and psychoeducation for treating posttraumatic stress disorder in an African refugee settlement. *Journal of Consulting and Clinical Psychology, 72*(4), 579-587.

Parker, R. G. (1995). Reminiscence: A continuity theory framework. *The Gerontologist, 35*(4), 515-525.

Pennebaker, J. W. (1989). Confession, inhibition, and disease. *Advances in Experimental and Social Psychology, 22,* 211-244.

Rappaport, J. (1995). Empowerment meets narrative: Listening to stories and creating settings. *American Journal of Community Psychology, 23*(5), 795-807.

Richeson, N., & Thorson, J. A. (2002). The effect of autobiographical writing on the subjective well-being of older adults. *North American Journal of Psychology, 4*(3), 395-404.

Salzer, M. S. (1998). Narrative approach to assessing interactions between society, community, and person. *Journal of Community Psychology, 26*(6), 569-580.

Schuster, E. (1998). A community bound by words: Reflections on a nursing home writing group. *Journal of Aging Studies, 12*(2), 137-147.

Smyth, J. M., Stone, A. A., Hurewitz, A., Kabell, A. (1999). Effects of writing about stressful experiences on symptom reduction in patients with asthma or rheumatoid arthritis. *Journal of the American Medical Association, 28*(14), 1304-1309.

Soltys, J., & Kunz, F. (2007). *Transformative reminiscence.* New York: Springer.

Vromans, L. P., & Schweitzer, R. D. (2011). Narrative therapy for adults with major depressive disorder: Improved symptom and interpersonal outcomes *Psychotherapy Research, 21*(1), 4-15.

Wang, D. (2011). Interdisciplinary methods of treatment of depression in older adults: A primer for practitioners. *Activities, Adaptation, and Aging, 35*(4), 298-314.

Wenzel, M., & Rensen, S. (2000). Changes in attitudes among children and elderly adults in intergenerational group work. *Educational Gerontology, 26*(6), 523-540.

Westcott, W. (1997). Picture writing and photographic techniques for the writing process. *The English Journal, 86*(7), 49-54.

Wright, J., & Chung, M. C. (2001). Mastery or mystery? Therapeutic writing: A review of the literature. *British Journal of Guidance & Counselling, 29*(3), 277-291.

Zalaquett, C., & Stens, A. (2006). Psychosocial treatments for major depression and dysthymia in older adults: A review of the literature. *Journal of Counseling & Development, 84*(2), 192–201.

Chapter 8: Dance as Internal Alchemy: The Healing Power of Expressive Movement

Emily Nussdorfer

"You can dance, not only to produce the union with yourself, or to manifest yourself, but in order to produce rain, or the fertility of women, or of the fields, or to defeat your enemy. The idea of an effect, of something produced, is always connected with the idea of dancing" (Jung, 1934, p. 46).

Introduction

The use of dance as an alchemical process to promote healing and integration of body, mind, and spirit has its roots in ancient indigenous traditions across the globe (Jung, 1934; Harner, 1990; Some, 1994; Katz, 1982). In these cultures, dance has been and still is used to celebrate individual and tribal identity, heal sickness, connect with guardian spirits or tribal ancestors, prepare for the hunt or war, bring prayers for good weather and prosperity, promote and celebrate rites of passage, weddings, and good crops, or facilitate tribal mourning (Jung, 1934; Harner, 1990; Some, 1994; Emerson, 1997; Katz, 1982; Gadon, 1989). In modern times, dance as a healing and empowering mode of self-expression, whether in practice or in therapy, is used by people of all ages, races/ethnicities and cultures, socio-economic backgrounds, genders and sexual orientations (American Dance Therapy Association [ADTA], 2001). Dance is used to relieve stress, promote physical vitality and strength, increase positive feelings (e.g., hope), build self-esteem, inspire romance and courtship, and promote self-expression, creativity, and insight (Roth, 1997; Halprin, 1995). Dance in therapeutic application and practice can provide a safe, nonverbal, physical channel for difficult emotions, helping people to release intense emotion and develop coping skills for challenging life circumstances. Dance is often used to bring people into positive, spontaneous, and playful connection with each other—diminishing isolation and building community spirit; it is especially effective with groups for the development of trust and rapport (Sandel, 1993). Dance can offer an individual a feeling of strength and liberation by supporting the authenticity of one's direct experience, and the integration of thought, feeling, and bodily experience in the present moment. Dance can express the ineffable essence of a person or a culture, effectively transmitting that meaning which cannot be communicated in words, but which longs to be expressed cathartically and symbolically in the body. Dance has been used with a variety of marginalized and challenged populations to support self-expression, build community spirit, and as a tool to promote social and personal change (Levy, 1992; ADTA, 2001).

This chapter explores how individuals, groups, and communities can experience healing, transformation, and empowerment through using dance expressively. The role of dance as a healing and empowering force by indigenous cultures is reviewed as well as its use as a way to sustain positive cultural identity for groups that have been historically marginalized or oppressed. An overview of dance movement therapy and the therapeutic applications of dance as an agent of personal healing and empowerment with various populations are provided. A project that combines therapeutic dance performance with other art forms is described. Designed to empower teen girls living in trauma-ridden environments, the program sought to advance their skills in order for them to become leaders and agents of change in their own lives and their communities. The chapter concludes with ethical considerations and tips for practitioners.

Dance Movement Therapy

Dance Movement Therapy (DMT) is broadly defined as "the psychotherapeutic use of movement as a process which furthers the emotional, cognitive, physical, and social integration of the individual" (ADTA, 2001). Dance as a form of therapy is expressive, physically integrative and inclusive. People of all ages, races/ethnicities, socio-economic backgrounds, genders, and sexual orientations can use dance. Participants may be struggling with a range of social, emotional, cognitive, or physical problems, including depression, trauma, grief, developmental disabilities, and behavioral/character disorders. People who want to improve the quality of their life and grow to their fullest potential also use DMT.

DMT is conducted in psychiatric hospitals and mental health centers, schools, juvenile detention centers and other correctional facilities, rehabilitation centers, homeless shelters, nursing homes, and corporate wellness programs. There are various schools and techniques of DMT, and also the way it is applied differs widely depending on the needs of the population being served (ADTA, 2001). Central to DMT is the transformative power of non-verbal communication and the tertiary process of creativity. The tertiary process, when applied during DMT, unfolds in three stages where 1) negative, seemingly self-destructive impulses and states of mind arising from the unconscious are 2) projected into a self-expressive, cathartic dance movement process, and 3) transform into a symbolic artistic experience accompanied by feelings of release, insight, and positive, new energies (Arieti, 1977; Johnson, 1998).

The Chacian Dance Therapy Technique

The Chacian DMT Technique, developed by the founder of the American Dance Therapy Association (Marian Chace) began as a transformative dance process that used movement as a tool for communication with institutionalized patients diagnosed with schizophrenia. The Chacian process helped patients come out of isolation and engage in healing, reality-based connections with others and themselves. This technique has since evolved into the main type of group DMT technique for both in-patient and community based groups for clients with a wide range of clinical problems (Chace, 1993; Chaiklin & Schmais, 1993).

The Chacian technique uses dance movement as the primary mode of interaction, communication, and expression. During a Chacian movement session, the use of rhythmic music is employed to meet group members where they are, both personally and culturally, to facilitate greater ease for self-expressive engagement in the dance movement process. When applying the technique, all movement directives of the therapist are based on nonverbal cues from the group members. During a Chacian group, the therapist guides movers through three progressive stages–warm up, mobilization/theme development, and closure–in such a way as to support the expansion of each movers' movement repertoire, while facilitating communal movement and interaction. The therapist supports group members' physical mobilization, organization, and emotional self-expression to encourage sustained engagement in movement, while expanding any symbolic actions that may arise in the group (Chaiklin & Schmais, 1993).

Central to the Chacian movement healing process is the concept of mirroring and kinesthetic empathy (Sandel, 1993). The mirroring process has the therapist mirror participants' movements to provide an empathic reflection of group members' unique expressions. This helps participants build trust and rapport with each other and the therapist on the nonverbal level. This in turn creates a safe container for the group, which allows symbolic imagery that may emerge in the dance movement process to be supported and utilized for individual and communal healing, self-expression, and catharsis (Sandel, 1993). The term kinesthetic empathy is defined as "the ability to accurately perceive, both on an intuitive and physiological level, a person's or a group's present emotional state, and to accurately reflect and empathically communicate to that person's or group's total psycho-physical experience using emotionally supportive, expressive and interactive movement" (Nussdorfer, 2010).

The dance movement therapist often chooses to use physical props to promote interaction and elicit expressive movement among members in the group and to help participants release movement inhibitions. Props are chosen for their effectiveness with particular populations and integrated into the three-part structure of any Chacian group; thus, they can be quite useful in developing themes and imagery. Examples of effective props for these purposes include balloons, stretch bands, various size balls, gym mats, parachutes, and scarves.

Dance Therapy in Therapeutic Application with Diverse Populations

Chacian DMT group can be used with a variety of different groups, including older adults suffering from depression and psychosis arising from cognitive impairment. The therapist may utilize light, colorful, interactive props–such as balloons or squishy balls–to initiate the group process. These props create a playful mood and elicit reflexive engagement. When combined with music from the era (e.g., 1940s and 1950s), the balloon toss turns into an expressive dance exchange, as therapist and patient hit the balloon in wide arcs, alternating with strength and lightness, reflecting the music. The therapist models dance moves and encourages expressive movement from the patients as they catch and throw this prop. The lightness and unpredictability of the balloon creates a sense of spontaneity and uplifts mood. This creative, interactional process not only promotes alertness and challenges patients out of lethargic, depressive states, but also encourages positive reminiscence by using music that is familiar and holds meaning for participants (Levy, 1992; Powers, 2013). After arousing the group via this playful technique, the therapist may then use deep breath work and more rhythmically mobilizing music to aide participants in stretching their bodies. The therapist will then guide participants through mobilizing movement sequences to promote cardiovascular health and stamina, weaving in periods of rest and reminiscence as needed. Props (e.g., scarves, parachute) are used to promote use of the full body, provide sensory stimulation, and continued engagement. The therapist will then facilitate closure, with gentle stretches and deep breaths—often using touch, hand holding, and communal songs to help participants slow down and integrate the moving experience. This process allows participants' bodies to cool down and relax while bringing group members together to reflect and share insights and experiences. The supportive and playful community spirit that is created through these healing dance interactions empower group members to feel supported and share personal stories and difficult feelings, while actively combating isolation and loneliness (Levy, 1992; Sandel & Hollander, 1995).

Moreover, the mobilizing and stress relieving dance movement processes allow the mind and body to focus, which promotes alertness and engagement. Through DMT, anxiety and confusion is pushed away, and positivity, relaxation, social connections, and support are built. Sadness or loss that emerged during the process is empathically supported, and positive memories are elicited to promote healing. During closure, participants often share that they feel that they have come together through the dancing and as a result feel happier.

When running a Chacian dance therapy group with autistic boys and girls, the therapist utilizes tools that support positive socialization, creative self-expression with impulse control, sequential movement processes that promote organization of body and mind, and increased focus (Erfer, 1995). For this young and exuberant population, the parachute is a wonderful tool to promote both containment and creative self-expression at the same time. The dance movement therapist may start by encouraging children to sit tightly and securely in their own piece of the parachute "pie." The therapist may draw upon the use of nursery rhymes and finger plays, such as the "itsy bitsy spider," to promote bodily organization and task focus. Or "ring around the rosy" can be used to build a strong sense of group rhythmic connection, promoting kinesthetic empathy and team skills. The therapist may choose uplifting and rhythmically organizing (e.g., Reggae) or soothing Irish ballads during the session to promote various movement qualities and rhythms. If the group is demonstrating exceptional self-containment and sharing, then the therapist may invite all group members to lift the parachute over their heads and form a tent, for example. Members are asked to imagine they are on a camping trip and to share an activity or help create a group story around the "campfire." These activities support both the containment and channeling of impulses; thus facilitating a structured release of pent up energy that is channeled into the free flow of imaginative self-expression, while at the same time fostering awareness of sharing movements, improving impulse control, and social skills (Erfer, 1995; Levy, 1992). Such a group will close with the same movement ritual used at the start and provide time for each child to share a favorite moment from the group experience.

Chacian group therapy sessions are adaptable to meet the needs of the participants. Using this approach with adolescent boys with severe behavioral disorders requires a different set of props and DMTprocesses to promote transformation and healing. Extreme hostility, emotional reactivity, and aggression are often accompanied by depression and hopelessness, which often arise from poor coping skills and exposure to ongoing traumatic situations (Harris, 2009; Johnson, 1987, 1998). Mistrust and resistance to engagement are common obstacles to overcome. Providing nonverbal means for a healthy channeling of aggressive impulses and developing spontaneous ways for members to address emotions, such as grief and depression, are equally important. The therapist must be skilled at watching the non-verbal behaviors of participants and be able to provide specific movement interventions that often include "going with the resistance" to facilitate trust and develop a therapeutic alliance. For example, the therapist may playfully ask members to "try to stay in the chair" as the therapist attempts to pull them up; this is a humorous device that uses resistance while simultaneously promoting engagement. Rather than asking them all to stand up, which gives them the opportunity to refuse, this technique allows for some playfulness that leads to compliance (Emunah, 1985). The therapist must create an environment that allows participants to feel that they will be met on their terms with their interests and passions honored and respected (Emunah, 1985; Duggan, 1995; Nussdorfer, 2010). The therapist should learn specific musical interests or favorite songs of group members as music is a central factor in developing a therapeutic alliance with adolescent populations. The therapist can then draw from this musical repertoire—utilizing different songs that support different kinds of rhythms (e.g., songs with grounding, organizing, mobilizing, or soothing rhythms; songs that speak to the emotional content present in the group; or songs that support the flow and release of emotional intensity). Furthermore, difficult emotional states are often suppressed so it is essential to meet participants where they are both in terms of music and movement to support cathartic release and promote awareness and new coping skills (Emunah, 1985; Johnson & Eicher, 1990; Johnson, 1998; Nussdorfer, 2010).

Empathically mirroring and providing a positive channel for participants' spontaneous nonverbal imagery, hostile gestures, or withdrawing movements can be expressed cathartically, symbolically, and even playfully through dance in the safety of the "arts play space" (Johnson, 1998). As nonverbal movement imagery emerges and is identified symbolically, the experience of the mover becomes archetypal and alchemical—insight and emotional liberation occurs. As participants experience release, they are able to share verbally what had been difficult to express to others. The group process may leave them feeling more supported by and supportive of their peers and more open to share aspects of themselves, which were difficult to express verbally.

Authentic Movement

Developed by Mary Whitehouse, Authentic Movement (AM) is a dance therapy process designed for individuals and groups that differs from the DMT Chacian technique in regards to the role of the therapist and participants. During a session, participants are asked to close their eyes and concentrate on feeling. Responding with movement to their inner impulses, participants allow any symbolic imagery and meanings to flow into their consciousness without censorship and respond to it with movement expression. In AM, the role of the therapist is to witness the mover in silence, only using the voice to prevent a participant from moving into another person or wall. The role of the mover is simply to respond "authentically" and feel the support of being witnessed by the therapist. Central to the transformational healing process is that of the therapeutic witness, both externally and within, and the alchemical process of working with the archetypal and symbolic aspects of the psyche to promote healing and empowerment. The goal of AM is to open up areas in the body that may contain buried emotions, which can occur over years of psychological patterning. These buried emotions need to be brought into consciousness so they can be released, transformed, and reintegrated. Verbal processing of the movement experience happens as needed after the session is completed. AM is used primarily with clients who have stronger ego boundaries than those in acute phases of psychological distress. Combining Jungian psychology with expressive movement, this approach helps individuals experience themselves "authentically" in response to their inner impulses. The process often promotes emotional catharsis, physical release, mind-body integration, and insight in movers (Levy, 1992; Adler, 2002).

Dance as an Expressive Therapeutic Practice

Many people are drawn to specific dance styles, such as jazz or hip hop or even fitness dance classes (e.g., Zumba), to learn dance skills and engage in an activity that is cathartic, health promoting, and empowering. Developing muscle knowledge and the movement repertoire of a particular dance technique, while releasing endorphins and developing physical fitness, also builds a sense of mastery, helps one feel more at home in one's body, provides a movement language for non-verbal self-expression, and improves both self-esteem and cognition (Powers, 2013; Chace, 1993). Through dancing as an expressive therapeutic practice, one can experience a sense of freedom, relief from stress and difficult emotions, and feel more empowered. A sense of community is also created as participants come together to learn and enjoy a particular dance form or style.

Group dance gatherings can include formal events such as *5rythyms, Contact Improvisation,* and *Journey Dance* or dancing around fire/drum circles or impromptu dance jams. These various types of group movement experiences bring people together to move in exploratory, spontaneous ways to experience a deeper connection to each other and to their bodies and to have the opportunity to utilize their physical bodies as vehicles of creative, artistic, spiritual, and emotional expression. Many people dance to feel the ecstatic physical experience of being alive and in motion as well as to develop physical fitness and health (Roth, 1997; Zehr, 2008). Others dance to experience emotional catharsis in their body, while accessing a deeper connection to the collective "body" of the universe (Roth, 1998; Adler, 1999). Some dance to "lose" themselves, and others dance to "find" themselves (Whitehouse, 1999a; Adler, 1999b; Chodorow, 1999; Roth, 1997; Halprin, 1995). Most dance connects the individual more deeply to themselves and others without the pressure of words.

During these moving group experiences, music or drumming plays a powerful part. Participants experience new ways of communicating with others, themselves, the elements, and the cosmos. These moving communications are at once more intimate and playful than regular verbal communications and also quite profound. Participants experience the depth of feeling embodied in self and community at the same time (Adler, 1999b). For some, engaging in learning and practicing a specific cultural dance style, such as flamenco, tango, or belly dance, is a way to deepen the self-exploration process by connecting to one's cultural roots and experiencing self-empowerment through this process (Smith, 2006). For others, trying on a new and exciting cultural experience can be liberating. An aspect of oneself that identifies with that culture's dance can find an outlet for expression.

Case Example: Dance Healing and Empowerment in Action: Reparative Education

This participatory dance performance project was held in a community center in Philadelphia. It was created as a way to facilitate a modern ritual of empowerment using dance with a group of adolescent, African American girls struggling with low self-esteem and self-destructive behaviors. Many were referred through juvenile court and behavioral health programs. The goal for this project was to use dance performance therapeutically in combination with mask creation to help each participant undertake an archetypal journey into the world of her imagination to identify sources of power and wisdom from within. Each girl would embody those qualities by creating and performing a "super girl" character who would dance her story of healing and transformation in full body mask in black light in front of an audience of family, friends, and supporters. Together the girls would dance a collective vision of change for their community and benefit from their community's support and witness.

The team included a trained masters level dance movement therapist (this author), who served as the project director/clinician, and three teaching artists in dance, theater/mime, and mask art making. All were chosen for their ability to establish a strong mentorship alliance with this population of girls through their art forms and personality.

The team met with the girls twice a week after school over the course of 12 weeks, and each session was approximately three hours. The team worked closely with the girls to help them find symbolic sources of inner strength through the art form of dance, combined with animal martial arts forms and yoga, creative visualization, mask making, character narrative, and mime. By the eighth week, participants had created character narratives that presented challenging aspects from their personal history, which had become symbolically transformed into healing powers. Each participant derived her super girl's character name from the unique healing power she discovered within herself as a result of overcoming personal obstacles. These names and stories naturally became archetypal and alchemical.

One such example is a participant, age 14, who created the character *The Healer*. In real life, a gang of girls had harassed her in her neighborhood for being "too pretty." In her story, a gang of girls attacked her, her face was cut, and blood ran down her dress. But she overcame this by healing herself with pink light and dancing away her pain. She used a pink scarf in her dance and combined movements of African samba with belly dance and encouraged the audience to clap in support of her dance. This participant had tremendous stage fright prior to performing, but shared that dancing in the mask made her feel safe and free. She wanted to help other girls who had been bullied know they could be free and powerful. Examples of other super girl character names were *the Leader*, *the Mother*, *Opticon Naturalle* (a Mother Nature figure), *the Peace Maker*, *Duality*, and *Conscience*.

The four-week rehearsal process was particularly vulnerable for some girls as deeper layers of grief, fear, and trauma emerged in the artistic process. Some girls began to act out, refused to rehearse, provoked arguments, or needed one-to-one support for redirection. Several shared fears about performing in front of an audience. The therapist and artists facilitated discussion circles encouraging participants to share their fears and draw strength from each other to cope with performance anxiety. Closing group with praise sessions was implemented to strengthen self-confidence and promote team spirit. During these sessions, the idea that their performance would only be as strong as the quality of support that each member gave to each other was emphasized as well as the importance of rehearsal to prepare for and overcome stage fright. Struggling through and learning the lessons of the rehearsal stage, allowed the girls to develop new skills of patience, perseverance, and collaboration. During this stage, one of the participants began to experience panic attacks and buried memories of past sexual abuse emerged. She was directed to appropriate venues of counseling and offered the choice to stop the choreography process; however, the participant expressed a desire to continue with the performance. She shared the following,

> "Going into the program, I had to deal with a lot of issues. I was having panic attacks and things like that from my past. But I could really open up and I could talk to Emily and I could talk to Mel and she had my back with anything… and all the girls, I learned from them, they just inspired me to keep moving. I feel great because I actually did something. I didn't need my mother or my father. I did it by myself. I don't know I probably would have gone crazy if I missed this opportunity. Now I have the sense that I can do anything. Things I used to be afraid of – I take it head on. I just can't describe it, it's an amazing feeling."

At the close of the project, participants shared feeling enhanced self-esteem and empowerment as well as appreciation for their peers. One participant declared that dancing was now her "getaway." She no longer needed to dream of going on vacation to relieve her stress. Another stated, "I think young girls my age need to be in programs like this…it changes who you are; just by being there together, just by showing up and creating together." This participant sums it all up: "a small group of girls can make an impact on Philadelphia."

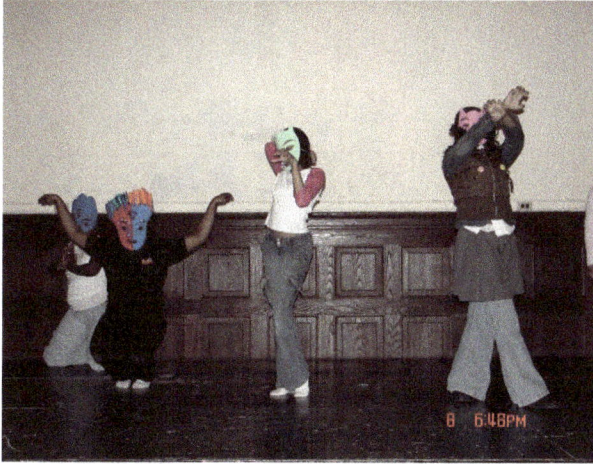

Title: *Animals developing their Super Girl characters*.
Location: Philadelphia, PA.
Photo by: Stephanie Zuckerman.

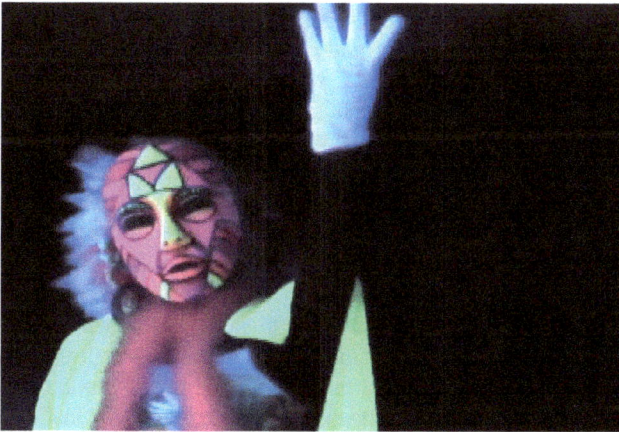

Title: *The Healer*.
Location: Philadelphia, PA.
Photo by: Still from video shot by Melody Vision.

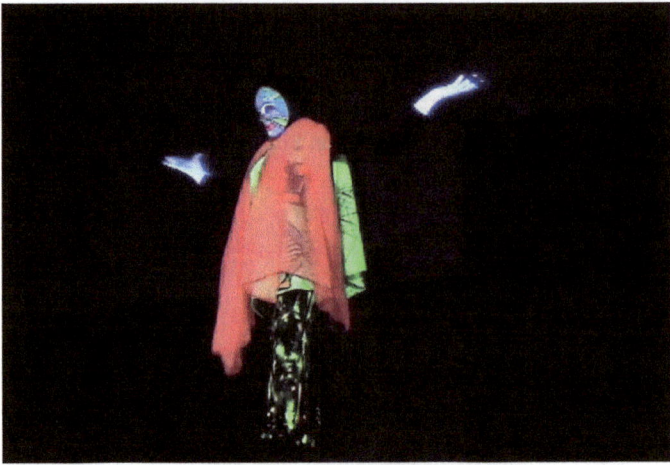

Title: *The Leader*.
Location: Philadelphia, PA.
Photo by: Still from video shot by Melody Vision.

Dance as a Cultural Healing Practice and Community Builder

Many indigenous cultures have drawn upon dance to promote the healing of physical, spiritual, and mental illness among tribal members as well as to empower and heal the collective (Chodorow, 1999; Jilek, 1974; Harner, 1990). One such culture is the Kung of Southern Africa's Kalahari Desert whose traditional hunter-gatherer way of life has been preserved for thousands of years. In their culture, dance is a central ritual around which the health and well-being of the entire tribe gravitates (Katz, 1982). For the Kung, healing is not just about curing illness; it is about growing physically, psychologically, and emotionally, both as an individual and a collective. The transformative dance process for the Kung is called the "long dance" and when collectively initiated by community members, commences at nightfall. Community members gather around a fire and begin to clap and sing to support the dancers. As the dancing progresses, some dancers feel a powerful burning sensation moving from the base of the spine to the bottom of the skull, which the Kung call "num" or "boiling energy." To access this "num" in such a way that it can then be shared with others as a source of healing and renewal, the dancer must undergo a "kia" or little death. Dancers undergoing "kia" often feel intense pain; many fall to the ground or faint or feel overwhelming fear. All must surrender to the "num" through "kia" so it can move through them as a healing force. Dancers then lay their hands on people to pull out physical illness or restore a troubled state of mind. The long dance brings the community together around one central purpose—healing and renewal. This collective dance process strengthens the community identity of the tribe, which can naturally become scattered by the demands of a nomadic life (Katz, 1982).

Dance in modern society can also function as a community builder. It may serve as a source of healing illness or as a way to empower and strengthen community identity. As members of a particular community come together to celebrate their cultural roots, they have an opportunity to mourn their losses, reconnect to cultural history and traditions, and experience the essence and soul of their culture. These cultural dance performances may also function as a bridge across cultural communities to bring a wider audience together around a particular expressive movement. Promoting the enjoyment of and understanding for a particular culture's dance expression can facilitate respect and support in the wider community. This in turn strengthens cross cultural community relationships and raises diversity consciousness.

Kulu Mele African Dance and Drum Ensemble, based in Philadelphia, PA, is one such company that serves to inspire and build community for the African Americans, while at the same time serving as a bridge to educate and inspire audiences from other cultural backgrounds. Kulu Mele's performance repertoire shares important cultural history, stories, myths, and traditions of the African Diaspora with audiences to educate and affirm African culture and experience. The dance company offers classes, workshops, and college residencies in African dance along with a youth outreach and development program that fosters cultural awareness and personal growth in the community. Building bridges of understanding, sustainability, and empowerment across and within cultural communities are the goals of Kulu Mele (Kulu Mele, 2013).

In sum, Kulu Mele, offers an approach that effectively educates others by witnessing and/or dancing the stories and myths that were considered vital to the essence of a culture and members of that cultural community experience a sense of empowerment (Jilek, 1974; Emerson 1997). Moreover, dance has been used to both express the experience and foster the empowerment amongst members of a marginalized/oppressed group, such as *Capoeira's* origins amongst the African slaves in Brazil (Almeida, 2007; Capoeira, 2002), the *Ghost Dance* phenomena of the Oglala Sioux (Neihardt, 2008), and *Breaking* in the United States (Schloss, 2009).

Benefits and Potential Challenges

Dance is versatile—it can be formal or informal. It can be used with anyone and includes every kind of movement. Dance can be a way to feel more liberated and empowered and can improve body image and self-esteem; however, because dance is based in the body, the experience of dancing, and even the concept of dance, can be challenging and even upsetting for people who have social shame linked to the idea of dancing. This may be especially challenging for those with limited movement, such as stroke victims, participants with physical disabilities, and those suffering from body image issues and/or disorders such as obesity, bulimia/anorexia, or those who are blind or hearing impaired (Fried, 1995). Nonetheless, dancing can be practiced effectively and supportively with eyes closed or open, in wheel chairs, on the floor, and even lying in a bed. There are so many ways to move expressively and cathartically to fully connect to one's physical and emotional experience. With appropriate therapeutic support, dance as an empowering form of self-expression and can be used as a way to develop strength, self-esteem, and improve mood for those who are struggling with physical limitations or body image issues. A sense of spontaneity and play is essential and can occur in any environment with the right music, props, and therapeutic skills and alliance.

Ethical Considerations

Clinical training in dance movement therapy at the master's level is a prerequisite for becoming a dance movement therapist. This training provides the practitioner with a strong foundation in psychotherapy with specialized training in DMT processes and techniques and clinical field experience. The dance movement therapist must have a thorough knowledge of dance and developmental body movement combined with an in-depth understanding of group therapy and role theory (Schmais, 1998).

The use of touch in therapy is always fraught with difficulty due to the potential for boundary confusion and/or violation, yet it is also a tremendously transformative force in DMT (Whitehouse, 1999). It is thus very important for the dance movement therapist to talk with the participant about how touch may be used in DMT and for what therapeutic purposes. Participants should be encouraged to share questions and concerns, and permission should be obtained from the participants. Ground rules around the use of touch in the dance therapy process should be established together. Prior to using touch, the dance therapist must discuss what touch means to the participant and establish how much, if any, would be helpful and supportive. For clients who have been physically or sexually abused, touch can be destabilizing or cause the psychic system to flood; however, for elders suffering from loneliness and depression, touch can be life sustaining (Levy, 1992; Sandel & Hollander, 1995).

When working with participants to develop a performance, it is important to get informed consent for photographs and publicity. Make sure each participant understands they have a choice to say no and not be photographed or not have their part of the performance used for publicity.

Tips for Practitioners

1. **Use dance as an adjunctive therapy to one's current practice.** Local clubs, organizations, or therapeutic groups can be found in many communities. Or if you are a skilled dancer, create your own recreational dance class.
2. **Be mindful of how music and props can be employed.** Both can be used to mobilize a participant's energy, help to ground and expand their movement repertoire, or serve as a catalyst to help develop symbolic imagery that may arise in the movement into conscious self-expression.
3. **The practitioner must build trust and establish a therapeutic alliance.** To do so, it is very important to be discerning about the appropriate movement interventions to use during the development of therapeutic goals. For example, if a participant is suffering from trauma or intense anger issues, it is important to move slowly into exploration of the body and to support grounding while providing safe channels for emotional discharge. For those participants struggling with psychosis or dementia, providing grounding and rhythmic activities that activate the core of the body, mobilizing all body parts sequentially, and promoting focus in the present moment is important, as is the focus on increasing interaction and decreasing isolation.

4. **Physical considerations.** The practitioner must be careful to help all participants learn to identify the difference between their physical comfort zone and their physical limits. It is important to identify if participants may have the tendency to push too hard or try for perfection with their bodies, which could result in injury. In these cases, the dance therapist must be very clear not to push too hard, but also be able to challenge the client to explore and move out of their comfort zone, which supports expansion of psychological range (Bartenieff & Lewis, 2002).

5. **Always meet the participant where they are in terms of movement.** Practitioners must be able to work with participants to help them identify their favorite movement patterns and areas of challenge as well as utilize music that the client is literally "moved" by. The therapist should empathically mirror and support a participant's movement. These actions support a strong therapeutic alliance and the participant's ability to trust and engage more deeply in their own journey through movement.

6. **Be aware of both your own and participants' cultural/personal movement biases.** The practitioner must do her/his own personal and cultural homework and be able to examine whatever bias s/he may be carrying physically. The DMT practitioner must be able to support the client in exploring her/his own cultural movement identity as may be appropriate for therapeutic goals.

7. **The dance therapist must be able to swiftly assess and monitor counter transference.** The dance movement therapist needs to be alert to participant's transference not only mentally and emotionally, but also physically and make choices as to how to use it therapeutically, on a moment-to-moment basis (Whitehouse, 1999).

8. **Consider having ongoing supervision in dance therapy.** This allows one to grow and develop your skills, which will support the psychophysical integration of your clients.

9. **As a practitioner, it is very important to take good care of your physical body.** Keep your core strong, your body flexible and in good health, your emotions flowing through your body, and your mind calm to best support your clients. Take time to nourish yourself with meditation, acupuncture, massage, and/or engage in Pilates/yoga classes in order to walk your talk with your clients. Be a role model of physical, emotional, and spiritual self-care.

10. **Dance for your own enjoyment!** Keep alive your passion for dance and expressive movement. Bring that playful passion and spontaneity into every session. Embody it and live it so that your clients will be inspired to explore, find, and express the enjoyment of fully inhabiting their own bodies.

Recommended Readings and Resources

American Dance Therapy Association. (2013). *Healing through movement*. Available at: www.adta.org.
Authentic Movement Community. (n.d.) *About Authentic Movement*. See:

www.authenticmovementcommunity.org/about.

Bartenieff, I., & Lewis, D. (2002). *Body movement: Coping with the environment.* New York: Routledge.

Halprin, A. (1995). *Moving toward life: Five decades of transformational dance.* Middletown, CT: Wesleyan University Press.

Levy, F. J. (1992). *Dance movement therapy: A healing art.* (Revised ed.). Reston, VA: American Alliance for Health, Physical Education, Recreation, and Dance.

Levy, F. J., Fried, J. P., & Leventhal, F. (Eds.). (1995). *Dance and other expressive art therapies: When words are not enough.* New York: Routledge.

Pallaro, P. (Ed). (1999). *Authentic movement.* Philadelphia, PA: Jessica Kingsley.

Sandel L., Chaiklin S., & Lohn, A. (Eds.). (1993). *Foundations of dance movement therapy: The life and work of Marian Chace.* Columbia, MD: The Marian Chace Memorial Fund of the American Dance Therapy Association.

References

Adler, J. (2002). *Offering from the conscious body: The discipline of authentic movement.* Rochester, NY: Inner Traditions.

Adler, J. (1999a). Body and soul. In P. Pallaro (Ed.), *Authentic movement* (pp. 160-189). Philadelphia, PA: Jessica Kingsley.

Adler, J. (1999b). The collective body. In P. Pallaro (Ed.), *Authentic movement* (pp. 190 – 204). Philadelphia, PA: Jessica Kingsley.

Almeida, P. (2007). *The essential guide to mastering the art.* London: New Holland.

American Dance Therapy Association. (2001). *What is dance movement therapy?* Retrieved from www.adta.org.

Arieti, S. (1977). New views of creativity. In F. F. Flach (Ed.), *Creative psychiatry* (pp. 3- 36). Ardsley, NY: Geigy Pharmaceuticals.

Bartenieff, I., & Lewis, D. (2002). *Body movement: Coping with the environment.* New York: Routledge.

Capoeira, N. (2002). *Capoeira: Roots of the dance-fight-game.* Berkley, CA: Blue Snake Books.

Chaiklin, S., & Schmais, C. (1993). The Chace approach to dance therapy. In S. L. Sandel, S. Chaiklin, & A. Lohn (Eds.), *Foundations of dance movement therapy: The life and work of Marian Chace* (pp. 75). Columbia, MD: The Marian Chace Memorial Fund of the American Dance Therapy Association.

Chace, M. (1993). Therapeutic concepts and techniques. In S. L. Sandel, S. Chaiklin, & A. Lohn (Eds.), *Foundations of dance movement therapy: The life and work of Marian Chace* (pp. 193 – 270). Columbia, MD. The Marian Chace Memorial Fund of the American Dance. Therapy Association.

Chodorow, J. (1999). Dance therapy and the transcendent function. In P. Pallaro (Ed.), *Authentic movement* (pp. 236-252). Philadelphia, PA: Jessica Kingsley.

Duggan, D. (1995). The "4s": A dance therapy program for learning disabled adolescents. In F. J. Levy, J. P. Fried, & F. Leventhal (Eds.*), Dance and other expressive art therapies: When words are not enough* (pp.225–240). New York: Routledge.

Emerson, N. (1997). *Unwritten literature of Hawaii: The sacred songs of the hula* (pp. 7–49). Honolulu, HI: Ai Pohaku Press.

Emunah, R. (1985). Drama therapy and adolescent resistance. *The Arts in Psychotherapy, 12,* 71-79.

Erfer, T. (1995). Teaching children with autism in a public school system. In F. J. Levy, J. P. Fried, & F. Leventhal. (Eds.), *Dance and other expressive art therapies: When words are not enough* (pp.191–211). New York: Routledge.

Fried, J.P. (1995). Sue and Jon: Working with blind children. In F. J. Levy, J. P. Fried, & F. Leventhal. (Eds.), *Dance and other expressive art therapies: When words are not enough* (pp.147-165). New York: Routledge.

Gadon, E. (1989). *The once and future goddess: A symbol for our time.* San Francisco, CA: Harper & Row.

Halprin, A. (1995). *Moving toward life: Five decades of transformational dance.* Middletown, CT: Wesleyan University Press.

Harner, M. (1990). *The way of the shaman* (3rd ed.). New York: Harper and Row.

Harris, D. A. (2009). The paradox of expressing speechless terror: Ritual liminality in the creative arts therapies' treatment of posttraumatic distress. *The Arts in Psychotherapy, 36*(2), 94-104

Johnson, D. R. (1998). On the therapeutic action of the creative arts therapies: The psychodynamic model. *The Arts in Psychotherapy, 25,* 85-99.

Johnson, D. R. (1987). The role of the creative arts therapies on the diagnosis and treatment of psychological trauma. *The Arts in Psychotherapy, 25,* 85-99.

Johnson, D., & Eicher, V. (1990). The use of dramatic activities to facilitate dance therapy with adolescents. *The Arts in Psychotherapy, 17,* 157–164.

Jung, C. G. (1934). A review of complex theory. In *The collected works of C. G. Jung* (vol. 8). Princeton: Princeton University Press.

Katz, R. (1982). *Boiling energy: Community healing among the Kalahari Kung.* Cambridge, MA: Harvard University Press.

Kulu Mele. (2013). *About Kulu Mele.* Retrieved from www.kulumele.org.

Levy, F. J. (1992). *Dance movement therapy: A healing art* (Rev. ed.). Reston, VA: American Alliance for Health, Physical Education, Recreation and Dance.

Neihardt, J. (2008). *Black elk speaks.* Albany, NY: State University of New York Press.

Nussdorfer, E. (2010). *Moving creation: A dance/movement and drama therapy-based program for preadolescent identity repair.* (Doctoral dissertation). Philadelphia, PA: Drexel University.

Powers, R. (2013). *Dancing makes you smarter.* Retrieved from: http://socialdance.stanford.edu/syllabi/smarter.htm.

Roth, G. (1997). *Sweat your prayers, movement as a spiritual practice.* New York: Jeremy P. Tarcher/Putnam.

Sandel, S. (1993). The process of empathic reflection in dance movement therapy. In S. L. Sandel, S. Chaiklin, & A. Lohn (Eds.), *Foundations of dance movement therapy: The life and work of Marian Chace* (pp. 98-111). Columbia, MD: The Marian Chace Memorial Fund of the American Dance Therapy Association.

Sandel, S., & Hollander, A. (1995). Dance/movement therapy with aging populations. In F. J. Levy, J. P. Fried, & F. Leventhal (Eds.), *Dance and other expressive art therapies: When words are not enough* (pp. 133-143). New York: Routledge.

Schloss, J. G. (2009). *Foundation: B-boys, b-girls, and hip-hop culture in New York.* New York: Oxford University Press.

Schmais, C. (1998). Understanding the dance movement therapy group. *American Journal of Dance Therapy, 20*(1), 23-35.

Some, M. P. (1994). *Of water and spirit: Ritual, magic, and initiation in the life of an African shaman* (p. 37-73). New York: Jeremy P. Tarcher/Putnam.

Smith, K. N. (2006). *Dance for development: Uyghur women in the Chinese diaspora creating self-empowerment through dance.* Paper presented at the 5th East-West Center International Graduate Student Conference, Honolulu, HI, USA.

Whitehouse, M. (1999). C. G. Jung and dance therapy: Two major principles. In P. Pallaro (Ed.), *Authentic movement* (pp. 73-101). Philadelphia, PA: Jessica Kingsley.

Whitehouse, M. (1999). The transference and dance therapy. In P. Pallaro (Ed.), *Authentic movement* (pp. 63-72). Philadelphia, PA: Jessica Kingsley.

Zehr, L. (2008). *The alchemy of dance: Sacred dance as a path to the universal dancer.* New York: iUniverse.

Chapter 9: The Rhythm of the Collective: Group Drumming as a Creative Arts Prevention and Intervention Strategy

Tina Maschi & Thalia MacMillan

Introduction

Group drumming, sometimes referred to as recreational music-making, is a creative arts intervention strategy that is gaining considerable attention because of its positive effects on individuals and groups. Specifically, this approach to practice can promote individual and collective well-being and empowerment (Maschi, MacMillan, & Viola, 2013). In recreational group drumming, participants sit in a drum circle or a group as they make music (Stone, 2005). Although the primary method of communication in group work is typically spoken language, the primary mode of communication in recreational drumming is singing and nonverbal communication; that is, individuals play percussion instruments (e.g., hand drums, tambourines, woodblocks, and shakers). Playing instruments places the intervention in the hands of the players as opposed to the use of music as therapy in which a trained expert is often required to administer the intervention (American Music Therapy Association, 1999). Group drumming is as an important and feasible creative arts intervention strategy in which the facilitator needs just a basic understanding of rhythm and hand drumming techniques to work with individuals, groups, and communities with varying musical skill levels.

It is also important to note that participation in the arts, including group drumming, is a basic human right (UN, 1949). Article 27 of the Universal Declaration of Human Rights (UDHR; UN, 1948) states that everyone has the right to freely engage in the cultural life of a community, enjoy the arts, and share in scientific advancement and its benefits. We assert that by providing individuals, families, and communities the opportunity to engage in the arts, such as group drumming, and having access to its research and evaluation findings about its effectiveness is a basic fundamental human right. If practitioners do not offer alternative modalities to their clients, then the arts are absent; thus, they are missing the opportunity to develop their clients full potential and provide them with alternative health care options. Consistent with a human rights approach, group drumming is a promising intervention for promoting health and well-being across the life course. The group drumming interventions reviewed here need further dissemination to other service settings and to other underserved and underrepresented populations, including incarcerated youth and adults. Advocacy at the institutional and legislative level should promote policies that infuse the arts as a core component of curriculum and health and social service settings.

This chapter examines group drumming as a creative arts intervention strategy that reduces stress and promotes healing, connection, and empowerment for diverse populations of clients and/or as a self-care strategy for professionals. The chapter is organized as follows: an overview of the benefits of group drumming is provided as well as the rationale for and description of the group drumming method. Next, a discussion of group drumming as an evidence-informed practice model, including a review of the relevant literature and the benefits and challenges when using group drumming as an intervention strategy are provided. We also provide an overview of our group drumming protocol called the *I-We Rhythm* program, which based on participants' feedback, was found to have had a curative effect as a type of "psychosocial spiritual" medicine. Ethical considerations are explored and tips for practitioners are detailed. Lastly, we provide recommended readings and resources for practitioners who want to further explore how to incorporate group drumming as a part of their practice toolkit.

Group Drumming: Description of the Method

The use of music has been shown to have positive intrapersonal and interpersonal outcomes among its participants. Studies on the use of music as an intervention have shown increased well-being, empowerment, group cohesiveness, and feelings of calmness and connectedness among diverse client populations (Bungay, 2010; Clift, Hancox, Morrison, Hess, Kreutz, & Stewart, 2010; Von Lob, Camic, & Clift, 2010). Diverse populations helped by music therapy include community members in good health (Bittman et al., 2001; Bungay, 2010; Clift et al., 2010; Olson, 2005), victims of trauma (Allen, 2001), individuals with terminal illnesses (Burns, 2001; Waldon, 2001), children, including those with developmental delays (Aldridge, Gustoff, & Neugebauer, 1995), at-risk adolescents (Keen, 2004; McFerran-Skewes, 2004), and individuals with mental health problems, including older adults (Hanser & Thompson, 1994; Lefevre, 2004). The purpose of group drumming is to empower individuals through the group experience and enhance well-being by reducing feelings of stress and tension in the individual. It allows the individual to use recreational drumming as a means to cope with issues that s/he may be experiencing.

Recreational drumming uses a group work modality; participants who take part in recreational drumming sit in a drum circle (Stone, 2005). Within the circle, the primary method of communication is singing or chanting (Clift et al., 2010). Other forms of nonverbal communication are utilized in recreational drumming as individuals play percussion instruments (e.g., hand drums, tambourines, woodblocks, and shakers). What is probably most useful about the approach is that it places the intervention in the hands of the players, as opposed to the use of music as therapy in which a trained expert is often required to administer the intervention (American Music Therapy Association, 1999). During the recreational drumming session a facilitator, who co-creates an environment with each of the participants, leads the group. In a recreational form of group drumming, making music through singing or percussion instruments is part of the therapeutic experience; it provides an opportunity for each participant to express her/himself in a unique way while allowing for active involvement in the group by each participant (Bungay, 2010).

The drum circle connects the individuals as they make music together, and it represents a shared collective and individualized experience (Clift, 2010; Hull, 1998). The positive impact of music has been documented among individuals in high-stress positions, such as health-care professionals and medical students (e.g., Bittman et al., 2004). Research on group drumming has also been shown to have positive outcomes, such as improving mood states and decreasing stress and job-related burnout among long-term health-care professionals and nursing students (Bittman, Bruhn, Stevens, Westengard, & Umbach, 2003, 2004, 2005; Bungay, 2010; Clift, 2010). Hands-on experiential group exercises, such as recreational group drumming, offer clients and professionals group-oriented stress management techniques that may reduce stress or burnout. For students in helping professions, who are in the budding stages of their careers, drumming provides another therapeutic tool or technique that they can use in their practice.

The art of group drumming must also be based in science to document positive outcomes and decrease the risk of unintended negative consequences that could adversely impact clients. One existing drumming program based in empirical evidence is the *Health RHYTHMS Group Empowerment Drumming Program*. The program uses the *Health RHYTHMS* protocol that consists of a series of 10-steps, which guide participants and facilitate communication and personal expression (Bittman et al., 2006). The program has four major learning objectives:

1. Understand the science of the mind-body connection in the context of music-making;
2. Become familiar with *Health RHYTHMS* protocol as a rhythm prescription for participants to benefit from active music-making;
3. Develop effective *Health RHYTHMS* group empowerment drumming facilitation skills;
4. Create and market integrated group drumming healthcare programs in the community.

Preliminary results of *Health RHYTHMS* program indicate that positive outcomes include reduction in stress and burnout rates, improvement in mood states, enhanced creativity, and bonding (Bittman et al., 2001). A link to this program is provided at the end of this chapter.

Group Drumming as a Self-care Strategy

The use of group drumming as a self-care strategy for professional social workers and other helping professionals is particularly important given the high stress situations that these professionals (as well as students studying in these areas) are exposed with regards to their workload and education. In light of studies that document job-related stress, job turnover (Barak, Nissly, & Levin, 2001), burnout (Jayaratne & Chess, 1984), secondary trauma (Bride, 2007; Dane, 2000; Nelson-Garedell & Harris, 2003), and mental health issues (Gold, 1998; Von Lob, Camic, & Clift, 2010) among social workers and other helping professionals, pursuing evidenced-based, self-care strategies including group drumming warrants further investigation. Based on recommendations from the literature, group drumming is conceptualized as consisting of three domains: inputs, process, and outputs, which are noted in effective drumming programs. Inputs for group drumming consist of the physical environment, the equipment, and the people who are involved. The process refers to the interaction with the instruments, and the outputs are the outcomes of the intervention (Bungay, 2010).

Inputs

According to Bungay (2010), the inputs for a group drumming circle consist of the actual physical space, the musical instruments, the group leader, and the participants who are involved in the process. These inputs are a critical aspect of the inner and outer workings that are needed for a drumming circle to function at its best. If the setting is not one where participants feel comfortable to express themselves, then the process and ultimately the outputs may be affected. Thus, having a space that is warm and welcoming is a essential to the success of the intervention. Most studies on group drumming have used a combination of a facilitator and music maker with varying levels of musical expertise. In some cases, the music maker was a professional musician (MacMillan, Maschi, & Tseng, 2012; Maschi & Bradley, 2010; Maschi et al., 2012), and in others, the music maker was someone trained in conducting group drumming sessions (Dickerson et al., 2012; Ho, Chinen, Streja, Kreitzer, & Sierpina, 2011; Stone, 2005). While this may seem inconsequential, the facilitator, who is the music maker of the group, is leading participants in music-making, and how comfortable they feel with the drumming or music-making influence the process.

The inputs of group drumming have been widely studied with diverse populations. Those helped by music include community members in good health (Bittman et al., 2001; Hoeft & Kern, 2007; Maschi & Bradley, 2010; Olson, 2005; Wachi et al., 2007), social work students (MacMillan et al., 2012; Maschi & Bradley, 2010; Maschi et al., 2012), mental health professionals (Ho, Chinen, et al., 2011a), victims of trauma (Allen, 2001), individuals with terminal illnesses (Burns, 2001; Waldon, 2001), pre-school children (Locke & Clark, 2009), children and those with developmental delays (Aldridge, Gustoff, & Neugebauer, 1995), patients during the prognosis stage of a chronic health problem (Kumar et al., 1999; Sahler, Hunter, & Liesveld, 2003), participants with chronic physical health conditions (Kumar et al., 1999; Sahler et al., 2003), at-risk adolescents (Clements-Cortes, 2013; Ho, Tsao, Bloch, & Zeltzer, 2011; Keen, 2004; McFerran-Skewes, 2004; Stone, 2005), soldiers with combat stress reaction or post traumatic stress disorder (Bensimon, Amir, & Wolf, 2008), and individuals with substance or mental health problems, including older adults (Blackett & Payne, 2005; Dickerson et al., 2012; Hanser & Thompson, 1994; Lefevre, 2004; Longhofer & Floersch, 1993).

Process

The group drumming process represents the group drumming participants' actual interaction with the instruments. It includes the inputs and the quality of the process of drumming, both of which strongly influence the intended outputs of the intervention (Bungay, 2010). The actual process of interacting with the music and creating a drumming circle is highly dependent on a multitude of factors, including the design of the recreational drumming protocol. The design of the protocol can be conceptual, cultural (Dickerson et al., 2012), or based in theory (Lee, 2001; MacMillan et al., 2012; Maschi et al., 2012). Those that are sensitive to culture or different aspects of theory have been found to be very effective (Dickerson et al., 2012; MacMillan et al., 2012; Maschi et al., 2012).

The protocol used in previous studies on recreational drumming varies widely. This may be related to feasibility issues, such as the type of population. The type of population may impact the process as it may need to be tailored to their specific needs. For example, working with pre-school children may denote that a shorter amount of time is needed to match the attentional issues of the children (Locke & Clarke, 2009). External factors related to the population may also impact the individual and group experience of drumming. For example, clients in a substance abuse facility who stay for a specific period of time (Blackett & Payne, 2005) or students enrolled in an eight-week course naturally limit the duration of the protocol (Maschi & Bradley, 2010; Maschi et al., 2012). The type of music-making, the number of individuals, and the amount of time for the protocol has the potential to impact the outputs. Most interventions described in the literature are a single session (Wachi et al., 2007) or training module consisting of participants who were in good health (Bittman, 2001; Ho et al., 2011a), but small groups (e.g., 6 or 7 individuals; Bensimon et al., 2008; Clements-Cortes, 2013) and larger groups (Ho, Chinen, et al., 2011b; Longhofer & Floersch, 1993; MacMillan et al., 2012; Maschi & Bradley, 2010; Wachi et al., 2007) have also been studied.

Outputs

Outputs refer to outcomes that were achieved as a result of participation in drumming (Bungay, 2010). Examples of outputs include the development or improvement of skills, such as learning to make music or enhancing social skills, and the improvement of biological and psychosocial well-being. Many drumming evaluations used qualitative methods to gather participants' feedback using open-ended questions about their perceived outcomes of the drumming intervention (Bungay, 2010; Clements-Cortes, 2013; Dickerson et al., 2012; Longhofer & Floersch 1993; Stone, 2005). While this may touch upon the quality of the process and outputs of drumming in group, other studies used the facilitator's responses to assess participants' experience of group drumming (Bungay, 2010; Clements-Cortes, 2013). The use of a facilitator as third party reporting may not be accurately representing the level of well-being actually experienced by participants.

Other group drumming programs used subjective and objective measures of well-being. The subjective measures have included the concept of well-being (Blackett & Payne, 2005; Ho et al., 2011b; Maschi & Bradley, 2010; MacMillan et al., 2012; Maschi et al., 2012; Wachi et al., 2007), self-esteem (Ho, 2011b), awareness (Locke & Clark, 2009; Maschi & Bradley, 2010; MacMillan et al., 2012; Maschi et al., 2012), engagement with others (Locke & Clark, 2009; Maschi & Bradley, 2010; MacMillan et al., 2012; Maschi et al., 2012), and social interactions (Kumar et al., 1999; Sahler et al., 2003; Silverman, 2009). The objective measures of well-being have included blood levels and genetic typing (Wachi et al., 2007). For example, studies using objective measures analyzed data from blood samples to examine physiological change in the neurological or immune systems as an indication of stress level (Bittman et al., 2001; Kumar et al., 1999).

The use of music to enhance well-being documents that group drumming has both positive internal and external outputs. Positive internal outcomes of group drumming, include increased well-being, reduced anxiety, increased feelings of calmness (as opposed to feeling stressed), and increased empowerment (Blackett & Payne, 2005; Ho et al., 2011b; Maschi & Bradley, 2010; MacMillan et al., 2012; Maschi et al., 2012; Wachi et al., 2007). Positive internal outcomes of group drumming have also included improved mood states, decreased stress and anxiety, decreased feelings of trauma, and decreased job related burnout (Bensimon et al., 2008; Bittman et al., 2003; Bittman et al., 2004, Bittman et al., 2005; Ho et al., 2011a; Wachi et al., 2007). This suggests that internal positive outcomes of well-being are multi-faceted and may be dependent upon the inputs and process.

Moreover, group drumming has been shown to have positive external outcomes, such as group cohesiveness and feelings of connectedness among diverse client populations (Dickerson et al., 2012; Locke & Clark, 2009; Maschi & Bradley, 2010; MacMillan et al., 2012; Maschi et al., 2012). Feeling connected to others or part of something may aid participants in feeling a higher sense of control over their experience. For example, Bensimon et al. (2008) used group drumming with soldiers who were experiencing a combat stress reaction. Prior to group drumming, the soldiers felt disconnected from others; however, post intervention, the soldiers felt more connected to others and felt a sense of belonging in the group (Bensimon et al., 2008). The use of group drumming enables communication to occur in a nonverbal domain in which all participants have an equal part as illustrated in the circle format and collective participation. Participants feel less judged because there is no right or wrong way to make a contribution. The use of group drumming for recreational purposes also demystifies the process to encompass everyone as opposed to the "trained and talented few." Most participants of drumming report a feeling of entrainment; that is, a state that encompasses feeling both calm and energized. Additionally the self-awareness of interpersonal and intrapersonal well-being, especially feelings of empowerment, connectedness, and community can assist individuals in translating these experiences to their lives to improve physical, mental health, social, and behavioral problems (e.g., Bittman et al., 2001; Silverman, 2006).

Case Example: The "I-We Rhythm" Program and Protocol

Based on the findings from the literature, we developed a program called the "I-We Rhythm" protocol, which was created for practitioners with minimal musical experience, particularly helping professionals. The *I-We Rhythm Program* was developed with considerations of inputs, process, and outputs for optimal group drumming experiences. Inputs for the workshop included the facilitator, the participants, and the environment. The protocol was facilitated by a licensed clinical social worker who is also a social work educator and a professional musician. The participants were master's level social work students who were taking part in a research course. To maximize the comfort level of the students, the environment was not the "normal" classroom associated with the course. Rather, the group drumming took place in a university lounge, which was more comfortable and private and had optimal lighting.

Conceptual Underpinnings

The conceptual underpinnings of the *I–We Rhythm* intervention are rooted in ecological-systems, empowerment/relational, and brain-based learning perspectives (Bronfenbrenner, 1979; Covington & Surrey, 1997; Jensen, 2000; Rose, 2000). A common thread among these perspectives is that external factors (e.g., the classroom environment) can influence students' ability to learn and feel empowered by their interactions with others in the classroom as well as reducing stress about the learning process. According to ecological systems theory, students are strongly influenced by their environment (Bronfenbrenner, 1979; Germain, 1979) and having social workers and students engage in group drumming has the potential to create a pseudo-contagion influence among the participants whereby they also want to play music. The empowerment perspective also provides a conceptual base for this intervention (Gutiérrez, Parsons, & Cox, 1998; Rose, 2000), which has been used with vulnerable populations as well as professionals (Frans, 1993). Empowerment refers to "skills in the exercise of interpersonal influence and the performance of valued social roles" (Solomon, 1976, p. 6), which has the advantage of decreasing feelings of powerlessness while increasing feelings of being energized (Gutiérrez & Lewis, 1999). The empowerment perspective is also consistent with some tenets of relational theory (Covington & Surrey, 1997), which suggests that healthy psychological development occurs through relationships that promote mutuality, cooperation, and a "power-with" approach. The opportunity to participate in a drumming circle may be characterized as a noncompetitive activity that promotes feelings of connectedness and cooperation with others (Belenky, Clinch, Goldberger, & Tarule, 1986; Covington & Surrey, 1997). Finally, brain-based learning informed this recreational music-making intervention given that this approach posits that students learn more effectively in a safe environment via multimodal teaching strategies (Caine, Nummella, Caine, & Crowell, 1999; Jensen, 1994). This form of learning can apply to the use of group drumming, because the student becomes an active participant in an activity that is often viewed as "fun." Therefore, students can feel less stress in an educational or agency environment. This approach also takes into account that every person has a unique learning style and, in this case, "a unique approach to playing the drum" (Jensen, 2000, p. 12).

Program Description

The *I–We Rhythm Program* begins with a two-hour introductory session that familiarizes participants with group drumming and its usefulness in practice with clients and as a professional self-care strategy. The session is divided into four segments: 1) introduction to recreational music-making as an intervention strategy; 2) the basics of rhythm; 3) introduction to percussion instruments and hand drumming techniques; and 4) participation in group drumming. A trained facilitator administers the program. Participants experience the "rhythm of social work" by learning the basics of rhythm and hand drumming techniques and then applying these skills in a series of group drumming exercises. The facilitator often provides the drums and hand percussion instruments, but participants are invited to bring with own. Group sizes generally range between 8 to 15 participants.

The facilitator's instrument toolkit includes a variety of hand drums (e.g., congas, djembes, and doumbeks) and hand-held percussion instruments (e.g., cowbells, agogo bells, wood blocks, tambourines, maracas, and other shakers). In addition to the hands-on experience with drumming, visual supports (e.g., handouts and PowerPoint slides) assisted participants in visualizing the basics of rhythm, rhythmic patterns, and hand-drumming techniques.

Verification of the I-We Rhythm Program

To determine the effectiveness of the program, participants' psychosocial well-being was evaluated before and after the group drumming activity. In order to maximize the analysis of the outputs, an exploratory pre-test/post-test study was conducted to examine the association between recreational drumming and well-being, including feeling tense/relaxed, stress/calm, energized, empowered, and connected (Maschi et al., 2012). It was hypothesized that participants would report lower levels of stress, an increase in feeling energized and empowered, and a greater connection with others. Similar to other drumming interventions, we found support that group drumming helped reduce stress and increase participants' psychosocial well-being and empowerment (Bittman et al., 2004; Burns, 2001; Levine & Levine, 1999; Longhoefer & Floersch, 1993; Maschi & Bradley, 2012; Maschi et al., 2012; Waldon, 2001).

Benefits and Potential Challenges

One of the primary benefits for both practitioners and participants alike is that the intervention does not require advanced musical expertise. This is an important aspect of this approach to practice given that music and music-making are powerful components of the human experience. Thus, music-making may represent another avenue to connect with clients, especially during group work. Group drumming also has a therapeutic effect, including for the facilitator. Improved well-being and decreased stress/burnout may be rewards that are reaped for the practitioner, which in turn, facilitates better practice with clients. Whether it used as an adjunctive technique with an individual or as a primary intervention for a group, the reduction in stress and improvement in well-being makes group drumming a good addition to the clinician's tool box.

Another benefit of group drumming is that it mainly uses nonverbal communication. This means that it can be used as an icebreaker activity to facilitate interaction among group members and build collective trust. Alternatively, it could be used as a way to communicate emotions without words. For example, people who have experienced difficult life experiences may find that group drumming offers a way to re-energize and connect with others without sharing, which can sometimes be a challenge. Furthermore, it also is a promising self-care strategy for reinforcing health and wellbeing among clients, students, and practitioners. If increasing well-being and empowerment is a key goal of an intervention, group drumming is a vehicle that practitioners can use to reach this goal.

There are surmountable challenges to the use of group drumming. One potential challenge is that the participants may not have ready access to percussion instruments. If this is the case, the practitioner can provide the instruments or perhaps seek out donations to purchase them, which could then be kept within the agency or facility for others to use. Participants may also be hesitant or anxious to drum because they do not feel they have the skills. Therefore, it is important for the facilitator to address anxiety and remind participants they do not have to be experts to participate in drumming. Facilitators can also ask participants about their level of experience with group drumming. In most cases, the majority of participants have no prior experience with drumming, and it puts the group members on equal footing being new to the drumming experience.

Ethical Considerations

Some key ethical considerations include access to instruments, boundaries issues, and the potential for drumming to evoke painful emotions among participants. First, access to instruments in the long-term could be an ethical issue—people could get excited about group drumming and find real benefits then not be able to afford one for use at home. Perhaps, used or second hand instruments could be found at thrift stores, pawn shops, or music stores that may be affordable for clients. If not, then a repurposed object may be a valuable stand-in, such as bucket or a small can filled with sand or pebbles. Second, boundaries amongst members may also be an issue. Music can provide a deep connection amongst people, and boundaries are always an issue when doing ongoing interventions with groups. Discussing this issue up front with group participants along with establishing ground rules may help thwart complicated situations. Practitioners should be aware of these issues and balance the need to maintain boundaries with client self-determination. Third, the drumming, chanting, or singing could trigger difficult or painful emotions for some. The practitioner needs to be sure that s/he is equipped to handle the situation. Much like other therapeutic practices, the release of emotion or painful experiences can create vulnerability for participants. The practitioner should be aware of resources in the community, including practitioners who may be available for individual therapy or emergency sessions that can be utilized if the practitioner is not already working with the client individually.

Tips for Practitioners

1. **How confident are you?** How confident are you at the following activities: leading a group, drumming, and facilitating of a drum circle? Will you need a co-facilitator? Do you need special permission within your agency to begin a new program or intervention? It is important to carefully consider your personal and agency needs prior to initiating a group drumming program.

2. **Who will participate in the group drumming intervention and in what roles?** Will the practitioner facilitate the group? Or will an external facilitator conduct the intervention? Will the practitioner be a participant? Are clients or staff able to choose whether or not they want to participate? The connection between inputs, process, and outputs is important to consider when planning the program or intervention.

3. **What kinds of drums will be used?** There are many percussion instruments that can be used for the intervention. One or more of the following can be used: hand drums, tambourines, woodblocks, and shakers. If it is possible, a range of instruments should be available for participants so they can chose the best way to express themselves during the music-making process. Participants may also want to use different instruments to express varying kinds of emotions. How will you get access to these instruments? Can you inform participants to bring their own instruments prior to the intervention, particularly if it is limited to one session?

4. **What are your expected outcomes?** Have you determined what outcomes you hope to achieve in a group drumming intervention? Do you hope to decrease stress or improve well-being, for example? How will you know when your goals have been achieved?

5. **Have you designed an evaluation plan?** How are you going to gather information about participants' experiences and the project outcomes, such as improved biological, psychological, and social well-being? Will you use quantitative and qualitative measures? How will you administer the measures? How will you analyze the information that was collected? For further information on evaluation, see Chapter 14, *Approaches to Evaluation: How to Measure Change when Utilizing Creative Approaches.*

6. **What are your future plans?** If the intervention proves helpful, have you considered a plan to continue a group drumming circle with participants who are interested? If yes, have you worked with the group to coordinate those plans? Have you considered obtaining funding? Many arts-based interventions, especially music, are fundable through local arts organizations. External funding may help you obtain the needed resources to run an ongoing group drumming program, including the purchase of instruments.

7. **Have you considered drumming as a method of self-care?** Given the high degree of burnout that can be found across helping professions, it is important to practice good self-care. Drumming may provide another method for practitioners who need time to re-energize.

8. **Have you considered a "train the trainer" option?** Drumming can be a source of self-empowerment, and group participants may want to become facilitators. Those participants who become trainers may experience further increase in self-confidence and well-being. Have you considered developing a training curriculum? A manual will help create consistency and organization for a training program, which can then also be used by others as the network of trainers grows.

9. **Have you considered developing your musical expertise?** As you develop your program over time, have you considered taking percussion lessons to learn the basic hand techniques and rhythm patterns on a particular instrument? Have you considered inviting professional drummers to participate in some group sessions to teach members basic rhythms? While group drumming interventions are not about professional music-making per se, increased musical training can be transferrable to participants, and the expertise of a professional musician may further encourage participants to pursue their passions.

10. **Have you considered holding a public event?** Many musical interventions often hold community concerts. Have you considered putting on a public event for participants to share their music with the community? The sharing process may have positive benefits for participants who gain experience and confidence through their public expression of creativity. For listeners, witnessing music-making can allow for the expression of personal emotions that are felt during this experience.

Recommended Readings and Resources

For a copy of the *I-We Rhythm* facilitator's guide, contact Tina Maschi at: tmaschi@fordham.edu.

Developmental Community Music. (2010). *Music with a mission.* Available at: http://drumcirclemusic.com/.

Remo. (2012). *HealthRHYTMS: Group empowerment drumming.* Available at: www.remo.com/portal/pages/hr/professional/healthrhythmsbasictraining. html.

Upbeat Drumming Resources. (2005). *Motivational drumming.* Available at: www.ubdrumcircles.com/online.php.

The Village Heartbeat. (2008). *Resources.* Available at: http://www.villageheartbeat.com/village-heartbeat-resources.php.

References

Aldridge, D., Gustoff, D., & Neugebauer, L. (1995). A pilot study of music therapy in the treatment of children with developmental delay. *Complementary Therapies in Medicine, 3,* 197–205.

Allen, K. (2001). Normalization of hypertensive responses during ambulatory surgical stress by perioperative music. *Psychosomatic Medicine, 63,* 487–492.

American Music Therapy Association. (1999). *About the music therapy association.* Retrieved from http://www.musictherapy.org/about.html.

Barak, M. E., Nissly, J. A., & Levin, A. (2001). Antecedents to retention and turnover among child welfare, social work, and other human service employees: What can we learn from past research? A review and metanalysis. *Social Service Review, 75*(4), 625–656.

Belenky, M. F., Clinch, B. M., Goldberger, N. R., & Tarule, J. M. (1986). *Women's ways of knowing.* New York: Basic Books.

Bensimon, M., Amir, D., & Wolf, Y. (2008). Drumming through trauma: Music therapy with post-traumatic soldiers. *The Arts in Psychotherapy, 35*(1), 34-48.

Bittman, B. B., Berk, L. S., Felten, D. L., Westengard, J., Simonton, C., Pappas, J., & Ninehouser, M. (2001). Composite effects of group drumming music therapy on modulation of neuroendocrine-immune parameters in normal parameters in normal subjects. *Alternative Therapeutic Health Medicine, 7,* 38–47.

Bittman, B. B., Berk, L., Shannon, M., Sharaf, M., Westengard, J., Guegler, K. J., & Ruff, D. W. (2005). Recreational music-making modulates the human stress responses: A preliminary individualized gene expression strategy. *Advances in Mind-Body Medicine, 11*(2), 31–40.

Bittman, B. B., Bruhn, K. T., Stevens, C., Westengard, J., & Umbach, P. O. (2003). Recreational music-making: A cost-effective group interdisciplinary strategy for reducing burnout and improving mood states in long-term care workers. *Advances in Mind-Body Medicine, 19*(3-4), 4-15

Bittman, B. B., Snyder, S., Bruhn, K. T., Liebfried, F., Stevens, C., Westengard, J., & Umbach, P. O. (2004). Recreation music-making: An integrative group intervention for reducing burnout and improving mood states in first year associate degree nursing students. *International Journal of Nursing Education Scholarship, 1*(1), article 12.

Blackett, P. S., & Payne, H. L. (2005). Health rhythms: A preliminary inquiry into group-drumming as experienced by participants on a structured day services program for substance-misusers. *Drugs: Education, Prevention, & Policy, 12*(6), 477-491.

Bride, B. E. (2007). Prevalence of secondary traumatic stress among social workers. *Social Work, 55,* 63–69.

Bronfenbrenner, U. (1979). *The ecology of human development: Experiments by nature and design.* Cambridge, MA: Harvard University Press.

Bungay, H. (2010). A rhythm for life: Drumming for wellbeing. *British Journal of Wellbeing, 1*(9), 13-15.

Burns, D. S. (2001). The effect of the bonny method of guided imagery and music on the mood and life quality of cancer patients. *Journal of Music Therapy, 38,* 51–65.

Caine, G., Nummela Caine, R., & Crowell, S. (1999). *Mindshifts: A brain- based process for restructuring schools and renewing education* (2nd ed.). Tucson, AZ: Zephyr Press.

Clements-Cortes, A. (2013). Health RHYTHMS: Adolescent drum protocol project with at-risk students. *Canadian Music Educator, 54*(3), 54-57.

Clift, S. (2010). Let the music play. *British Journal of Wellbeing, 1*(1), 15–17.

Clift, S., Hancox, G., Morrison, I., Hess, B., Kreutz, G., & Stewart, D. (2010). Choral singing and psychological wellbeing: Quantitative and qualitative findings from English choirs in a cross national survey. *Journal of Applied Arts and Health, 1*(1), 19–34.

Dane, B. (2000). Child welfare workers: An innovative approach for interacting with secondary trauma. *Journal of Social Work Education, 2*(2), 27–38.

Dickerson, D., Robichaud, F., Teruya, C., Nagaran, K., & Hser, Y. I. (2012). Utilizing drumming for American Indians/Alaska Natives with substance use disorders: A focus group study. *American Journal of Drug and Alcohol Abuse, 38*(5), 505-510.

Frans, D. J. (1993). A scale for measuring social worker empowerment. *Research on Social Work Practice, 3*(3), 312–328.

Germain, C. (Ed.). (1979). *Social work practice: People and environments— An ecological perspective.* New York: Columbia University Press.

Gold, N. (1998). Using participatory research to help promote the physical and mental health of female social workers in child welfare. *Child Welfare, 77*(6), 701–724.

Gutiérrez, L., Parsons, R., & Cox, E. (1998). *Empowerment in social work practice: A sourcebook.* Pacific Grove, CA: Brooks/Cole.

Hanser, S. B., & Thompson, L. W. (1994). Effects of a music therapy strategy on depressed older adults. *Journal of Gerontology, 49,* 265–269.

Ho, P., Chinen, K. K., Streja, L., Kreitzer, M. J., & Sierpina, V. (2011a). Teaching group drumming to mental health professionals. *Explore: The Journal of Science and Healing, 7*(3), 200-202.

Ho, P., Tsao, J. C. I., Bloch, L., & Zeltzer, L. K. (2011b). The impact of group drumming on social-emotional behavior in low-income children. *Evidence-Informed Complementary and Alternative Medicine,* Article ID 250708, 1-14.

Hoeft, L., & Kern, P. (2007). The effects of listening to recorded percussion music on well-being: A pilot study. *Canadian Journal of Music Therapy, 13*(2), 132–147.

Hull, A. (1998). *Drum circle spirit: Facilitating human potential through rhythm.* Reno, NV: White Cliff Media.

Jayaratne, S., & Chess, W. (1984). Job satisfaction, burnout, and turnover: A national study. *Social Work, 29*(5), 448–453.

Jensen, E. (1994). *The learning brain.* San Diego: Brain Store.

Jensen, E. (2000). *Brain-based learning.* San Diego, CA: Brain Store.

Keen, W. A. (2004). Using music as a therapy tool to motivate troubled adolescents. *Social Work in Health Care, 39*(3/4), 361–373.

Kumar, A. M., Tims, F., Cruess, D. G., Mintzer, M. J.,. Ironson, G., Loewenstein, D., Cattan, R., & Kumar, M. (1999). Music therapy increases serum melatonin levels in patients with Alzheimer's disease. *Alternative Therapies in Health and Medicine, 5*(6), 49–57.

Lee, J. (2001). *The empowerment approach to social work practice (2nd ed.).* New York: Free Press.

Lefevre, M. (2004). Playing with sound: The therapeutic use of music in direct work with children. *Child & Family Social Work, 9,* 333–345.

Levine, S. K., & Levine, E. G. (Eds.) (1999). *Foundation of expressive arts therapy: Theoretical and clinical perspectives.* Philadelphia: Jessica Kingsley.

Locke, K., & Clark, D. (2009). Can African drumming impact the social/emotional development of young children? *Canadian Children, 34*(2), 10-15.

Longhofer, J., & Floersch, J. (1993). African drumming and psychiatric rehabilitation. *Psychosocial Rehabilitation Journal, 16*(4), 3–11.

MacMillan, T., Maschi, T., & Tseng, Y. F. (2012). Measuring perceived well-being after recreational drumming: An exploratory factor analysis. *Families in Society: The Journal of Contemporary Social Services, 93*(1), 74-79.

Maschi, T., & Bradley C. (2010). Recreational drumming: A creative arts intervention strategy for social work teaching and practice. *Journal of Baccalaureate Social Work, 15*, 53-66

Maschi, T., Macmillan, T., & Viola, D. (2013). Group drumming and well-being: A promising self-care strategy for social workers. *Arts & Health: An International Journal for Research, Policy, and Practice, 5*(2), 142-151.

McFerran-Skewes, K. (2004). Using songs with groups of teenagers: How does it work? *Social Work with Groups, 27*(2/3), 143–157.

Nelson-Garedell, D., & Harris, D. (2003). Child abuse history, secondary traumatic stress, and child welfare workers. *Child Welfare, 82*(1), 5–26.

Olson, K. (2005). Music for community education and emancipatory learning. *New Directions for Adult & Continuing Education, 107,* 55–64.

Rose, S. M. (2000). Reflections on empowerment-based practice. *Social Work, 45*, 403–412.

Sahler, O. J. Z., Hunter, B. C., & Liesveld, J. L. (2003). The effect of using music therapy with relaxation imagery in the management of patients undergoing bone marrow transplantation: A pilot feasibility study. *Alternative Therapists in Health and Medicine, 9*(6), 70–74.

Silverman, M. J. (2009). The effect of single-session psychoeducational music therapy on verbalizations and perceptions in psychiatric patients. *Journal of Music Therapy, 46*(2),105–131.

Solomon, B. (1976). *Black empowerment: Social work in oppressed communities.* New York: Columbia University Press.

Stone, N. N. (2005). Hand-drumming to build community: The story of the Wittier Drum Project. *New Directions for Youth Development, 106,* 73–83.

United Nations (1948). *Universal Declaration of Human Rights.* New York: Author.

Von Lob, G., Camic, P., & Clift, S. (2010). The use of singing-in-a-group as a response to adverse life events. *International Journal of Mental Health Promotion, 12*(3), 45–53.

Wachi, M., Koyama, M., Utsuyama, M., Bittman, B. B., Kitagawa, M., & Hirokawa, K. (2007). Recreational music-making modulates natural killer cell activity, cytokines, and mood states in corporate employees. *Med Sci Minit, 13*(2), 57-70.

Waldon, E. G. (2001). The effects of group music therapy on mood states and cohesiveness in adult oncology patients. *Journal of Music Therapy, 38,* 212-238.

Chapter 10: Horticultural Therapy: The Art of Growth

Keith A. Anderson & Jennie R. Babcock

"The glory of gardening: hands in the dirt, head in the sun, heart with nature. To nurture a garden is to feed not just the body, but the soul." -- Alfred Austin

"My hoe as it bites the ground revenges my wrongs, and I have less lust to bite my enemies. In smoothing the rough hillocks, I smooth my temper." --Ralph Waldo Emerson

Introduction

Throughout history, horticultural activities (e.g., gardening, cultivation) have provided more than simply nourishment. As far back as 2000 BC, people-plant interactions have been linked with a wide range of therapeutic benefits—soothing the soul, feeding the spirit, and inspiring the mind (Jellicoe & Jellicoe, 1995). Indeed, the power of horticulture as both an art form and a "healing art" is documented in the writings of the ancient Egyptians, Greeks, and Romans (Albers, 1991). Beginning in the 1800's, horticulture was viewed as an accepted clinical practice or treatment for mental illness and was used as therapy for patients suffering from mania and other psychiatric maladies. The 20th century saw the establishment of the first horticultural therapy education programs in the United States and the professionalization of this discipline (American Horticultural Therapy Association [AHTA], 2012; Relf, 2006). Currently, horticultural therapy is a widely accepted modality to treat various mental health issues, to enhance physical and social functioning, and to improve quality of life for a variety of populations.

The goals of this chapter are to provide information on horticultural therapy and expand the common understanding of "art" and "artful interactions" as well as inspire creativity in practice. This chapter explores and explains the definitions, theory, process, and practice of horticultural therapy as a healing art.

The literature and research on horticultural therapy is reviewed in terms of the impact and effect on four primary groups: children, individuals with physical and mental health challenges, incarcerated populations, and older adults. Gaps in our understanding of horticultural therapy and limitations in extant research are also discussed along with ethical considerations for practitioners. Finally, an overview of an innovative horticultural therapy program is presented along with tips for practitioners.

Definitions and Theoretical Underpinnings of Horticultural Therapy

As horticultural therapy has developed, definitions have flourished. Broad definitions include any form of people-plant interaction, including social horticulture (e.g., recreational gardening, community gardening) and nature-assisted therapy (e.g., wilderness therapy, outdoor adventure therapy). While there are undoubtedly benefits to these activities, more recent definitions of horticultural therapy have become more focused, providing a more structured approach to implementing therapeutic interventions. This more structured definition moves us away from the oversimplified notion that, "if it's horticulture, it's therapy" and allows for systematic evaluation and the development of evidence-based practices (Relf & Dorn, 1995). For the purpose of this chapter, we use the following definition of horticultural therapy:

> Horticultural therapy is a professionally conducted client-centered treatment modality that utilizes horticulture activities to meet specific therapeutic or rehabilitative goals of its participants. The focus is to maximize social, cognitive, physical and/or psychological functioning and/or to enhance general health and wellness (Haller, 2006a, p. 5).

There are several theories that have guided the development and support for the use of horticultural therapy. In "attention-restoration theory," Kaplan and Kaplan (1989) posit that humans use involuntary attention in natural environments and directed attention in urban and artificial environments. Involuntary attention is theorized to be the least stressful since the brain is wired to react more effectively and easily to the organic visual patterns of the natural world. Directed attention requires individuals to process stimuli that are foreign to the brain leading to stress and impaired functioning. Natural environments and interactions allow individuals to escape the routine and thoughts of the "daily grind" and to experience attention without labor, which fosters a sense of fascination and relaxation.

Closely related, psycho-evolutionary theory suggests that humans react positively to plants and nature due to our evolutionary development in the natural environment. The sights, sounds, and textures of nature are part of our fiber, and therefore, we react positively to these stimuli. The stress and busyness of the modern, artificial world can overload our senses, creating feelings of hyper-arousal and anxiety. A return to the simplicity of the natural environment restores balance and reduces stress. Research has largely supported this theory, including studies where physical healing has been enhanced for patients simply by having a window with a view of nature (Ulrich & Parsons, 1992).

Learning theory has also been applied to help explain the impact of nature on well-being. This perspective holds that individuals adapt to and find comfort in environments that are linked to their own upbringing (Ulrich, 2000). In other words, culture and environment influences preferences, feelings of security, and a sense of home. For instance, an older adult in a nursing home who grew up on a farm may find pleasure in growing vegetables in a facility garden. This theory is more person-centered than the evolutionary perspective and focuses on the lived experiences of the individual. An interesting counter-point to this theory is that it does not account for the generally positive responses that individuals have to nature regardless of their background or past experiences (Relf, 1992). Perhaps the three perspectives presented here, taken in combination, can best account for the potential benefits of nature and horticultural therapy.

Elements and Types of Horticultural Therapy

The process of horticultural therapy generally consists of three main elements– clients, defined treatment goals, and treatment activities (Relf & Dorn, 1995). Clients include individuals and groups diagnosed with a specific challenge, disability, or need. Clients can include those with psychiatric issues, physical disabilities, intellectual and developmental disabilities, educational issues, and those facing social and environmental challenges. Clients served by horticultural therapy are also diverse in terms of age, ability, and situation, such as school children, prisoners, hospitalized and institutionalized individuals, and older adults. Each group presents unique needs, challenges, and opportunities to benefit from horticultural therapy.

Defined treatment goals include both facility goals and individual/client treatment goals. Facility goals may include "vocational rehabilitation and return to the community at reduced functional level, maintenance of functional level without institutionalization, sheltered or supported employment, and delayed progress of disability" (Relf & Dorn, 1995, p. 100). For instance, horticulture therapy might be used with an adult with an intellectual disability whose anxiety is impacting her/his activities in a sheltered workshop. Individual treatment goals are often related to facility to goals, but are driven by the individual and are person-centered. For example, a person with a substance abuse issue may achieve their goal of sobriety through the use of horticultural therapy. It is critical to note that these goals are achieved through written and actionable objectives. This allows for professionals to monitor progress, adjust treatment strategies, and evaluate and document evidence-based practices.

The third element of horticultural therapy, treatment activity, is designed to help individuals and facilities to meet their goals. As previously noted, broad definitions of horticultural therapy allow for the inclusion of activities such as sitting in a meditation garden, taking nature walks, and participating in outdoor recreation. More structured definitions of horticultural therapy (such as the one used in this chapter) strongly encourage the use of living plants in treatment activities. Examples of these treatment activities include gardening clubs in residential group homes, intergenerational community garden programs, potted plant care in retirement and nursing homes, and school gardens for children. It should be noted that the involvement and direction of a trained professional (e.g., horticultural therapist, activities therapist, or social worker with specialized training) is essential in treatment activities (Haller, 1998). In developing horticultural therapy treatment activities, professionals should also consider the following: 1) activities should be designed to be "the smallest, simplest one available to achieve the desired goal, thus benefiting the most clientele (Relf & Dorn, 1995, p. 101); and 2) the activity is the therapy and the end result is not necessarily indicative of success or failure–essentially, the treatment activity "is only a tool in the therapeutic process, not the end goal" (Catlin, 2006, p. 39).

There are four general types of horticultural activities: horticultural therapy, therapeutic horticulture, vocational horticulture, and social horticulture (AHTA, 2012). As previously reviewed, horticulture therapy involves clients and trained therapists seeking to achieve specified goals. Horticultural therapists typically have professional training and registration. While some horticultural therapists hold degrees in this discipline, individuals from other disciplines (e.g., social work, nursing, activities professionals) are also capable of facilitating interventions with additional training. Therapeutic horticulture is similar to horticulture therapy in that clients use plants and activities, yet differs as goals are not clinically defined and the facilitator may not have specialized training in horticulture therapy. Both horticultural therapy and therapeutic horticulture programs are employed in health care settings (e.g., hospitals, rehabilitation facilities) and residential settings (e.g., nursing homes, group homes). Vocational horticulture trains individuals to find employment in the horticulture industry, such as working in nurseries, grounds keeping, landscaping, and small-scale farming. Vocational horticulture is commonly offered to adults with intellectual and developmental disabilities, incarcerated individuals, and at-risk youth. Social horticulture is far less structured than the other three programs. As the title implies, the goal is socialization and recreation and typically includes community gardening and garden clubs. Specific goals and outcome measures are not generally recorded in social horticulture. Horticultural activities with specific groups will be discussed in the next several pages. Examples of evidence-informed interventions that have been shown to be effective will also be presented for each group.

Horticultural Therapy with Specific Populations

Children

In 2013, it was estimated that 50 million children were enrolled in primary and secondary public schools in the United States. Another five million were enrolled in private schools (National Center for Education Statistics, 2013). It is well-documented that childhood is an impressionable life stage and that the knowledge, attitudes, and behaviors in childhood have life-long ramifications. As such, horticultural therapy and activities with children have the potential for lasting effects. Horticultural therapy and activities can be divided into two categories: general and "targeted" programs. General programs typically focus on school gardens with the goal of experiential learning and social skill building. Targeted horticultural therapy programs focus on specific issues, conditions, and challenges, such as intellectual and developmental disability and illness (e.g., cancer, cerebral palsy). (Note: Horticultural therapy programs for youth involved in the corrections system are briefly reviewed later in this chapter.)

School gardening programs range in type and scope (for a review, see Blair, 2009). These include projects using in-ground gardens, raised beds, potted plants, ponds, butterfly gardens, and composting. The goals of gardening programs vary from learning about environmental and nutritional issues to improving academic performance and increasing emotional and social well-being. Unfortunately, the impact of school gardening programs is not well-researched. This is not to suggest that school gardens are ineffective in helping children grow, quite the contrary. School gardening programs can improve test scores and reduce behavioral issues as well as serve as interactive vehicle to learn about environmental nutritional issues. Given the prevalence of obesity and diabetes in the general population, school gardens may be more valuable in the coming years.

Targeted horticultural therapy programs engage children dealing with specific issues. While some targeted programs use gardening activities similar to school gardens, other programs provide one-on-one therapy. The goals of targeted horticultural therapy program with children are to improve physical functioning, emotional status, and social skills. The body of literature on targeted horticultural therapy programs is quite limited; however, in initial testing, several programs do appear to show benefits. For instance, one structured horticulture program found increased sociality in children with intellectual disabilities (Kim, Park, Song, & Son, 2012). Other targeted programs have provided anecdotal evidence of effectiveness, yet findings were non-significant. Additional research in this area is needed for the field to move forward.

Taking a closer look at a recent novel study, researchers designed a horticultural therapy program to evaluate the impact of a school garden on children's knowledge, preference, and consumption of fruits and vegetables (Parmer, Salisbury, Shannon, & Stuempler, 2009). Second grade classes were divided into three groups: 1) nutrition education and gardening; 2) nutrition education only; and 3) a control group (i.e., educational programming as usual). The goal was to determine which intervention was most effective in encouraging healthy eating knowledge and behavior. Results indicated that the nutrition education and gardening group gained greater nutritional knowledge than the control group and demonstrated higher levels of preference and consumption of fruits and vegetables. As previously discussed, such interventions have great potential to instill healthy eating habits that may follow children throughout their lives.

Mental Health

In any given year, over 25% of the adult population in the United States suffers from a mental health condition, and approximately 6% of the adult population suffers from serious mental illness. These mental health conditions include clinical depression, anxiety disorders, bipolar disorder, attention deficit/hyperactivity disorder, eating disorders, schizophrenia, and personality disorders. Contrary to common thought, mental health disorders are the leading cause of disability in the United States (National Institute of Mental Health, 2014).

As previously mentioned, natural environments and horticultural activities have long been used to comfort those with mental health disorders. Today there is a small but growing body of compelling evidence that horticulture therapy and activities can have therapeutic benefits for clients suffering from a variety of mental health disorders.

A range of horticultural therapy interventions have been developed and used to address mental health issues. These include the use of flower and vegetable gardening, passive interactions with nature (e.g., walking through gardens, watching flora and fauna), education on gardening and nutrition, and harvesting and cooking projects. These horticultural therapy interventions are commonly combined with other treatment modalities (e.g., pharmacological treatment, individual and group therapy) as part of an overall treatment strategy. Recent research has found that horticulture therapy interventions for individuals suffering from mental illness can offer relief from stress, interrupt negative ruminations, improve mood, reduce the severity of symptoms, facilitate social interaction, and improve overall well-being (Adevi & Martensson, 2012; Barley, Robinson, & Sikorski, 2012; Gonzalez, Hartig, Patil, Martinsen, & Kirkevold, 2010; Gonzalez, Hartig, Patil, & Martinsen, 2011; Grabbe, Ball, & Goldstein, 2013). While promising, there are considerable limitations to our knowledge regarding horticultural therapy and mental health, most notably, understanding the complementary effect of horticultural therapy with more traditional treatments.

A recent study involving horticulture therapy and activities for individuals with clinical depression provides a good example of how this complementary treatment modality can be both feasible and beneficial (Gonzalez et al., 2010; Gonzalez et al., 2011). Participants diagnosed with clinical depression took part in a 12-week horticultural therapy program that involved planting, potting, and cultivation on local farms. There was also a passive component to the intervention that involved observing the fields and gardens and listening to the sounds of nature. The researchers found that symptoms of depression decreased consistently across the 12 weeks of the intervention and remained significantly lower three months after the conclusion of the study. A decrease in rumination (i.e., brooding over one's problems) also occurred, and participants reported that the intervention "contributed to change in my view of life" (Gonzalez et al., 2011, p. 76). As shown in this study, horticulture therapy can be effective in addressing mental health issues and should be considered as society seeks cost-effective and alternative ways to address these widespread problems.

Corrections

The Bureau of Justice Statistics (2013) reported that almost seven million adult offenders were involved with the correctional system in 2012. One in every 35 adults was on probation, parole, or incarcerated–a sobering statistic that illustrates the magnitude of this issue. With resources spread thin and a focus on punishment, rehabilitation opportunities for this population tend to be few. Despite this trend, horticultural therapy and activities have been used in corrections settings (primarily prisons) as a form of both rehabilitation and vocational training over the past 20 years. Research on the types of programs that are effective is sparse, as are the long-term impacts of horticultural therapy in terms of behavior modification, recidivism, and vocational success.

Several types of horticultural therapy and activities have been developed and evaluated with incarcerated individuals and ex-offenders (i.e., individuals on parole), including men, women, and youth. In correctional facilities, prison gardens are the most common. Some prison garden programs provide simple opportunities for people-plant interaction, while others are more structured and include trained facilitators with specific goals and measured outcomes. Early studies of structured horticultural therapy in prisons found that participants experienced positive changes in self-esteem and self-confidence (Rice & Remy, 1998), less vulnerability to addiction (Richards & Kafami, 1999), social skill building and improved problem solving (Flagler, 1995), and life satisfaction (Migura, Whittlesey, & Zajisek, 1997). Programs that focused on vocational horticulture were found to have mixed results. Some offenders and ex-offenders benefitted from improved job skills and greater control over their lives (O'Callaghan, Robinson, Reed, & Roof, 2010). Other vocational horticulture programs found few differences between youth offenders in horticultural-focused probation programs and traditional programs in terms of recidivism and emotional well-being; however, gains were observed in job skills, paying restitution and fines, and benefits to the community (e.g., landscaping, cleaning, and beautification; Cammack, Waliczek, & Zajicek, 2002). Clearly, more research is needed to help elucidate the effectiveness of horticultural therapy in correctional settings.

The Prison Master's Gardeners program is an example of a promising horticultural therapy intervention in the correctional setting (O'Callaghan et al., 2010). Educators from a university extension program designed, implemented, and evaluated a 72-hour horticulture course at a women's prison. Information was presented to participants regarding site preparation and planning, planting, irrigation, pruning and maintenance, harvesting, and job training in the horticulture field. The goals of the program were behavior modification and vocational readiness. Analyses of quantitative and qualitative data indicated that the horticulture program was related to high levels of self-responsibility, interpersonal skills, and self-responsibility and work. Participants also noted positive behavior change (e.g., lower levels of drinking post-incarceration, healthier lifestyles) and improved job skills. Unfortunately, it remains to be seen whether wide-spread use of horticultural therapy in corrections settings will be available in this era of cost-cutting and privatization of prisons.

Older Adults

The Census Bureau (2013) has projected that the population of older adults (i.e., those age 65 and older) will more than double from 43 million in 2012 to 92 million in 2060. As the population continues to grow older, it is anticipated that there will be an even greater need for therapies and approaches that complement or even replace pharmacological interventions. Horticultural therapy shows great promise in filling this role. It has been used with older adults for several decades, and researchers have begun to establish a considerable body of literature on the benefits of people-plant interactions. In particular, a number of studies have focused on older adults with dementia–a growing concern for families and society. Older adults are thought to be particularly amenable to the benefits of horticultural therapy as they are vulnerable to physical limitations, social isolation, and institutionalization (i.e., nursing home placement). Horticultural therapy is designed to address these issues by increasing social interaction, encouraging introspection, and experiencing fascination and connection with the natural world.

As reported in several recent reviews, a range of people-plant interactions and activities has been examined in terms of their impact on older adults. These include social horticulture, such as gardening, and horticultural therapy activities, such as structured interventions using people-plant interactions to address issues such as depression, anxiety, and adjustment to nursing home placement. One systematic review reported that "the majority of studies found some evidence that gardening is enjoyable for older adults and that it benefits overall quality of life, physical ability, and activeness" (Wang & MacMillan, 2013, p. 175). For example, studies found that horticultural activities were related to decreased pain, greater physical strength and flexibility, improved coordination, and improved ability to perform activities of daily living. Another study found improvements in social interaction and self-confidence (for a review, see Wang & MacMillan, 2013). For older adults with dementia, horticultural activities have been found to be related to high levels of social interaction and participation in activities, overall well-being, and emotional affect (for a review, see Gonzalez & Kirkevold, 2013).

A good example of a horticultural therapy intervention with older adults with dementia can be found in the work of D'Andrea, Batavia, and Sasson (2007-2008). The goal of their 12-week intervention was to delay cognitive decline and consisted of a range of activities that appealed to the diverse physical and cognitive abilities of participants, including: "planting seeds, observing the seedlings, watering existing plants, repotting new seedlings in bigger containers, and picking dead leaves out of the pots and plants" (pp. 11-12). A trained therapeutic recreation specialist facilitated the intervention. At the beginning of each session, the facilitator described the project, encouraged participants to select the activities that interested them most, assisted and encouraged participants, and led discussions to enable participants to talk about the activity. When compared with a control group, participants in the intervention were found to have significantly higher levels of cognitive functioning. These types of programs have great promise, especially considering the option for long-term interventions for those living in institutions or regularly attending community-based programs (e.g., adult day services).

Conclusion

Horticulture has a long, rich history as a healing combination of art and science. Encountering the natural world through horticultural activities provides opportunities to learn, share, and experience wonder, fascination, and transcendence. Over the past several decades, horticultural activities have been used to treat a wide range of issues and populations, and horticultural therapy has grown to be an accepted treatment modality. While research has begun to demonstrate the potential feasibility and effectiveness of horticultural therapy, more rigorous research is needed to further our understanding of this promising treatment option. In the future, we may find that the garden is more than simply a plot of land–it is a place of artful self-expression, personal growth, and holistic healing.

Case Example: Bonsai Therapy with Older Adults

In the following section, details on a horticultural therapy intervention for older adults in a nursing home setting are provided. This specific intervention has not yet been implemented and tested, but the authors have developed this intervention with the hopes that an opportunity for its application will occur. Older adults have been found to be at high risk for social isolation, depression, and anxiety, and these conditions can lead to elevated rates of morbidity and mortality (Centers for Disease Control, 2008). For older adults living in nursing home settings, these mental health issues can be amplified as they leave their homes and are surrounded by strangers and unfamiliar and often sterile environments. Horticultural therapy interventions have the potential to help older adults adjust to nursing home placement and to reduce their risk of social isolation. In the following paragraphs, we discuss the use of bonsai plants in horticultural therapy and detail the structure and format of this intervention.

Bonsai is the ancient Japanese art of cultivating and shaping small trees in containers. Bonsai is an expression of creativity filled with a sense of wonder and contemplation. It also provides growers with opportunities to engage in a living and growing art project (Koreshoff, 1998). The bonsai therapy intervention proposed here is an 8-week program specifically designed for nursing home residents. The goals of the intervention are to help older adults adjust to the nursing home environment and to increase socialization. The intervention has three components: education, activity, and reflection. During each one-hour session, participants will 1) learn about the bonsai tree and techniques for bonsai care; 2) implement techniques (e.g., potting, pruning, watering); and 3) reflect upon their own bonsai trees and share their work with others. The intervention is tailored to the abilities of each participant and assistance will be provided to those with limited capacities. A trained facilitator will implement the intervention.

While the intervention will vary according to the activity of the day, the following is an example of a typical session. The session starts by gathering all participants into a defined space. It is important to try to eliminate outside distractions during the intervention, so a separate, quiet space within the facility should be selected. In this session, the educational component focuses on techniques for pruning the bonsai trees. The facilitator will review the rationale for pruning and introduce and demonstrate the tools and techniques used in this process. Showing pictures or short videos on pruning can also be useful in educating participants. The participants will then implement these techniques using their own bonsai trees during the next 20 to 30 minutes. It is important that the facilitator takes a hands-on approach and works with each participant individually. Over-pruning a bonsai tree can be problematic, and participants should be encouraged to be judicious and intentional with their pruning. In the final 15 minutes, the participants will present their bonsai trees to the group and discuss their pruning decisions and their reactions to the intervention. The facilitator will then wrap up the session, remind participants of the upcoming session, and reiterate the instructions for caring and watering the bonsai trees between sessions. Participants will then take their bonsai trees with them to their rooms and care for them until the next session. (Note: Facilitators should schedule an additional 10-15 minutes for those sessions when data is to be collected.)

A structured pre- and post-intervention measurement schedule will be used to gauge the impact of the bonsai therapy intervention on social isolation, emotional well-being, and personal growth. Outcome measures will be administered to participants prior to beginning the intervention, at the conclusion of the intervention, and one month following the conclusion of the intervention. The following scales are suggested to measure each of the variables under consideration for this intervention:

- *Social Isolation* – The six-item Friendship Scale will be used to measure social isolation. Sample items include: "I had someone to share my feelings with" and "I felt alone and friendless (reverse scored)." This scale is valid and reliable as well as easy to administer and score (Hawthorne, 2006).
- *Emotional Well-Being* – The 15-item Geriatric Depression Scale–Short Form will be used to measure emotional well-being. Sample items include: "Are you in good spirits most of the time?" and "Do you feel your situation is hopeless?" This scale is widely used and has been found to be reliable and valid (Sheikh & Yesavage, 1986).
- *Personal Growth* – The seven-item Personal Growth subscale of Ryff's Psychological Well-Being Scale will be used to measure participants' sense of development. Sample items include: "For me, life has been a continuous process of learning, changing, and growth" and "I am not interested in activities that will expand my horizons (reverse scored)." This scale has been used with older adults and is valid and reliable (Ryff & Keyes, 1995).

Our approach to studying the effects of bonsai therapy would provide a way to increase the knowledge base regarding the use of horticulture in practice. We encourage other practitioners to make use of some or all of the plan proposed here or create other horticultural therapy interventions that make use of the research process. Sharing these findings in publications and presentations is also essential to spreading information regarding the many benefits of horticultural therapy.

Benefits and Potential Challenges

As we have seen, horticultural therapy and activities can have a variety of benefits and may be effective in improving the well-being and quality of life of a number of groups in society. Summarizing the benefits from a research perspective is challenging given the relatively small number of studies that have evaluated horticultural therapy and the wide variability in methods and application. Examining the goals of horticultural therapy interventions may provide some clarity. For illustrative purposes, these goals have been collapsed into three categories–education, socialization, and treatment.

Education appears to be one of the areas in which horticultural therapy has the greatest potential. As we have seen, educating children on the process of growing food and on nutrition can have a positive impact on choosing and consuming healthy food. Horticultural therapy interventions aimed at diabetes and diet knowledge for adults have also been found to be effective (Lombard et al., 2013). Moreover, the educational goal of horticultural therapy may benefit adults, as we have seen in vocational horticulture programs in correctional settings.

Socialization is also an important goal of horticultural therapy programs, and benefits can be seen in children, adults, and special populations. For example, children can learn social skills, adults with depression can reduce feelings of social isolation, and older adults with dementia can experience a feeling of inclusiveness through horticultural therapy activities.

The final goal, treatment effectiveness, has less empirical support and is a much "heavier lift" for horticultural therapy. Issues such as depression, autism, schizophrenia, addictions, and criminal behavior can be deeply rooted problems, and questions remain as to the long-term benefits that horticultural therapy can provide. However, research does suggest that horticultural therapy can be beneficial as part of an overall treatment strategy. Multidimensional problems typically require multidimensional approaches, and horticultural therapy should be considered in the care planning for these complex issues.

Certain challenges exist in the implementation of horticultural therapy activities. While horticultural therapy has gained credibility in the past few decades, it is still often viewed as an "alternative treatment" approach. Getting buy-in can be a challenge and may require educating clients and families and lobbying facility administrators. Although costs are typically low, those associated with building gardens, facilitating interventions, and providing supplies are still a consideration. Agencies and facilities will be required to allocate some funding for these expenses, which can be a challenge. Closely related is reimbursement for horticultural therapy, which is currently not widely provided by insurance providers (including Medicare/Medicaid). This is problematic in terms of revenue generation–a very real consideration for most agencies and facilities. In the future, this barrier may erode as the research on horticultural therapy continues to grow.

Ethical Considerations

There are very few ethical considerations or concerns due to the relatively benign nature of horticultural therapy. For practitioners, the first ethical consideration lies in selecting participants for the intervention. Inclusion and exclusion criteria should be fair and clearly specified. When there are limitations in the number of participants, individuals should be provided with alternatives. For example, a school with space for a small garden may need to limit participation in a horticulture therapy program. Rather than excluding interested students, it might be best to set up an alternating schedule or to incorporate elements that do not require direct interaction with the garden (such as a classroom education component). The length of the horticultural therapy intervention could pose another ethical issue for practitioners. Horticultural therapy interventions are often time-limited. Participants should be made fully aware of the length of the intervention and be prepared for termination. Therapists should visit this topic early and continuously with participants to prevent disappointment or other negative emotions following the conclusion of the intervention.

Protecting participants also raises the issue of safety and "doing no harm" (i.e., the ethical principle of nonmaleficence). Horticultural therapy often involves the use of sharp and potential dangerous tools. In the case of offenders in correctional settings, these tools can be used as weapons and strict monitoring and control must be in place prior, during, and after the horticultural intervention. Children with behavioral issues can pose the same danger and teachers should closely monitor access to and use of gardening tools. Finally, adults with cognitive deficits (e.g., individuals with dementia and intellectual disabilities) may harm themselves or others with these tools due to confusion or agitation. Practitioners should allocate tasks and tools based upon their understanding of each participant's ability and emotional stability.

Tips for Practitioners

1. **Seek out training**. Training opportunities through continuing education, mentorship, and workshops, which is available both in-person and online, is necessary for implementing horticultural therapy. Interested practitioners should refer to the American Horticultural Therapy Association website for an updated list of training programs (see http://ahta.org/).

2. **Consider horticultural therapy as an adjunctive intervention to current practice**. For example, in outpatient settings, perhaps a client could care for a small, easy plant (e.g., African Violet) or one that grows quite large, but is still easy to maintain, such as a peace lily. Alternatively, an herb garden could be started on an inpatient unit with new residents taking over where the discharged clients left off. Moreover, the plants could also be used as a metaphor during regular therapeutic sessions as a way to explore growth and essential needs.

3. **The dual benefits of horticultural therapy lends well to non-therapeutic settings.** For example, it can be used with children in schools for both educational as well as social needs, including cooperation. Alternatively, it could be beneficial on a medical rehabilitative unit where patients stay in residence for a number of weeks or months. As their healing proceeds, they can focus on the care of a plant or garden with other residents of the facility.

4. **It is critical to establish a treatment plan based upon an assessment of the client and/or group.** The treatment plan includes identifying overall goals and specific objectives, developing an intervention plan (including the means of measuring progress and outcomes), initial development of the horticultural intervention, plans for documenting progress and outcomes, and plans for the termination phase of the

intervention (Haller, 2006b). This plan will help the practitioner implement the intervention/activities and monitor change in participants.

5. **Be innovative when suggesting a horticultural program to administration.** For example, when making a pitch for a composting program at a prison, consider highlighting the fact that composting cuts waste by recycling garbage, which in turn is good for the environment and a cost savings approach for the prison. Moreover, composting gives those who are incarcerated a positive activity that is skill building and the soil could be sold for a small cost to prison employees and others, which could then be used to support the program or other programs within the prison.

6. **Horticultural activities should match the needs of participants and the goals of the intervention.** Horticultural therapy activities can include (but are not limited to) cultivating, potting, pruning, harvesting, education on gardening and nutrition, and nursery operations. It is important to remember that the activities are the tools for treatment (Catlin, 2006). Practitioners should also be cognizant of the fact that participants often have different backgrounds, needs, and abilities. Activities should be tailored to meet the needs and abilities of each participant (Catlin, 2006).

7. **Collect data when implementing horticultural therapy.** To further develop the field and the practice, additional research is essential (see Chapter 14 for information regarding research). This is also a likely requirement when seeking funding as those who invest in "alternative" programs want to know that the money is well spent.

8. **Documentation is critical across each phase of the horticultural therapy intervention.** Progress notes document the process of the intervention, facilitate replication, and help assessment of fidelity to the treatment plan. Manualizing the intervention can also help others who wish to evaluate and replicate the intervention (Sieradzki, 2006).

9. **Horticultural therapy interventions are meant to be enjoyable and growth-oriented activities.** Practitioners should enjoy both the preparation and implementation of the interventions and convey this sense of joy to participants. Some potential participants may be reluctant to join horticultural therapy programs or fail to initially see the benefits of such activities. An enthusiastic, supportive, and high-spirited approach can help with recruitment and contribute to the overall success of the intervention.

10. **Celebrate the results of a horticultural therapy program.** This can also be beneficial for participants as well as fulfilling for practitioners. Showcases and open-houses to display the fruits of participants' labor are wonderful ways to cap off an intervention. They are also powerful vehicles for garnering support from facility administrators and from the community at large.

Recommended Readings and Resources

American Horticultural Therapy Association. (2013). *Advancing the practice of horticulture as therapy*. Available at: http://ahta.org.

Haller, R. L., & Kramer, C. L. (Eds.). (2006). *Horticultural therapy methods: Making connections in health care, human service, and community programs.* Binghamton, NY: Haworth Press.

Jiler, J. (2006). *Doing time in the garden: Life lessons through prison horticulture.* Oakland, CA: New Village Press.

Marcus, C. C., & Sachs, N. A. (2014). *Therapeutic landscapes: An evidence-based approach to designing healing gardens and restorative outdoor spaces.* Hoboken, NJ: John Wiley & Sons.

Marshall, M., & Pollock, A. (Eds.). (2012). *Designing outdoor spaces for people with dementia.* Sydney, Australia: Hammond Press.

Simson, S. P., & Straus, M. C. (1998). *Horticulture as therapy: Principles and practice.* Binghamton, NY: Haworth Press.

References

Adevi, A. A., & Lieberg, M. (2012). Stress rehabilitation through garden therapy: A caregiver perspective on factors considered most essential to recovery. *Urban Forestry & Urban Greening, 11*, 51-58.

Albers, L. H. (1991). The perception of gardening as art. *Garden History, 19*(2), 163-174.

American Horticultural Therapy Association. (2012). *Definitions and positions.* Retrieved from: http://ahta.org/sites/default/files/DefinitionsandPositions.pdf.

Barley, E. A., Robinson, S., & Sikorski, J. (2012). Primary-care based participatory rehabilitation: Users' views of a horticultural and arts project. *British Journal of General Practice*, e127-e134.

Blair, D. (2009). The child in the garden: An evaluative review of the benefits of school gardening. *Journal of Environmental Education, 40*(2), 15-38.

Bureau of Justice Statistics. (2013). *Correctional populations in the United States, 2012.* Retrieved from www.bjs.gov/index.cfm?ty=pbdetail&iid=4843.

Cammack, C., Waliczek, T. M., & Zajicek, J. M. (2002). The Green Brigade: The psychological effects of a community-based horticultural program on the self-development characteristics of juvenile offenders. *HortTechnology, 12*(1), 82-86.

Catlin, P. A. (2006). Activity planning: Developing horticultural therapy sessions. In R. L. Haller & C. L. Kramer (Eds.), *Horticultural therapy methods: Making connections in health care, human service, and community programs* (pp. 33-58). Binghamton, NY: Haworth Press.

Centers for Disease Control. (2008). *The state of mental health and aging in America.* Retrieved from www.cdc.gov/aging/pdf/mental_health.pdf.

D'Andrea, S. J., Batavia, M., & Sasson, N. (2007-2008). Effect of horticultural therapy on preventing the decline of mental abilities of patients with Alzheimer's type dementia. *Journal of Therapeutic Horticulture, 18*, 8-17.

Flagler, J. S. (1995). The role of horticulture in training correctional youth. *HortTechnology, 5*, 185-187.

Gonzalez, M. T., Hartig, T., Patil, G. G., Martinsen, E. W., & Kirkevold, M. (2010). Therapeutic horticulture in clinical depression: A prospective study of active components. *Journal of Advanced Nursing, 66*(9), 2002-2013.

Gonzalez, M. T., Hartig, T., Patil, G. G., & Martinsen, E. W. (2011). A prospective study of existential issues in therapeutic horticulture for clinical depression. *Issues in Mental Health Nursing, 32*, 73-81.

Gonzalez, M. T., & Kirkevold, M. (2013). Benefits of sensory garden and horticultural activities in dementia care: A modified scoping review. *Journal of Clinical Nursing.* Published online first at http://onlinelibrary.wiley.com/ doi/10.1111/jocn.12388/pdf.

Grabbe, L., Ball, J., & Goldstein, A. (2013). Gardening for the mental well-being of homeless women. *Journal of Holistic Nursing, 31*(4), 258-266.

Haller, R. L. (1998). Vocational, social, and therapeutic programs in horticulture. In S. P. Simson & M. C. Straus (Eds.), *Horticulture as therapy: Principles and practice* (pp. 43-70). Binghamton, NY: Haworth Press.

Haller, R. L. (2006a). The framework. In R. L. Haller & C. L. Kramer (Eds.), *Horticultural therapy methods: Making connections in health care, human service, and community* programs (pp. 1-22). Binghamton, NY: Haworth Press.

Haller, R. L. (2006b). Goals and treatment planning: The process. In R. L. Haller & C. L. Kramer (Eds.), *Horticultural therapy methods: Making connections in health care, human service, and community* programs (pp. 23-32). Binghamton, NY: Haworth Press.

Hawthorne, G. (2006). Measuring social isolation in older adults: Development and initial validation of the Friendship Scale. *Social Indicators Research, 77*, 521-548.

Jellicoe, G., & Jellicoe, S. (1995). *Landscape of man* (2nd ed.). London: Thames & Hudson.

Kaplan, R., & Kaplan, S. (1989). *Experience in nature: A psychological perspective.* Cambridge: Cambridge University Press.

Kim, B. Y., Park, S. A., Song, J. E., & Son, K. C. (2012). Horticultural therapy program for the improvement of attention and sociality in children with intellectual disabilities. *HortTechnology, 22*(3), 320-324.

Koreshoff, D. (1998). *Bonsai: Its art, history, and philosophy.* Portland, OR: Timber Press.

Lombard, K. A., Beresford, S. A. A., Ornelas, I. J., Topaha, C., Becenti, T., Thomas, D., & Vela, J. G. (2013). Healthy gardens/healthy lives: Navajo perceptions of growing food locally to prevent diabetes and cancer. *Health Promotion Practice.* Published online first at http://hpp.sagepub.com/content/early/2013/07/09/1524839913492328.full.pdf.

Miguera, M. M., Whittlesey, L. A., & Zajicek, J. M. (1997). Effects of a vocational horticulture program on the self-development of female inmates. *HortTechnology, 7*(3), 299-304.

National Center for Education Statistics. (2013). *Projections of education statistics to 2021.* Retrieved from

http://nces.ed.gov/programs/projections/projections2021/tables/table_01.
asp.

National Institute of Mental Health (2014). *The numbers count: Mental disorders in American.* Retrieved from http://www.nimh.nih.gov/health/publications/the-numbers-count-mental-disorders-in-america/index.shtml#Intro.

O'Callaghan, A. M., Robinson, M. L., Reed, C., & Roof, L. (2010). Horticultural training improves job prospects and sense of well-being for prison inmates. *Acta Horticulturae, 881,* 773-778.

Parmer, S. M., Salisbury-Glennon, J., Shannon, D., & Struempler, B. (2009). School gardens: An experiential learning approach for a nutrition education program to increase fruit and vegetable knowledge, preference, and consumption among second-great students. *Journal of Nutrition Education and Behavior, 41*(3), 212-217.

Relf, P. D. (1992). Human issues in horticulture. *HortTechnology, 2*(2), 159-171.

Relf, D., & Dorn, S. (1995). Horticulture: Meeting the needs of special populations. *HortTechnology, 5*(2), 94-103.

Relf, D. (2006). Agriculture and health care: The care of plants and animals for therapy and rehabilitation in the United States. In J. Hassink & M. van Dijk (Eds.), *Farming for health* (pp. 309-343). Netherlands: Springer.

Rice, J. S., & Remy, L. L. (1998). Impact of horticultural therapy on psychosocial functioning among urban jail inmates. *Journal of Offender Rehabilitation, 26*(3/4), 169-191.

Richards, H. J., & Kafami, D. M. (1999). Impact of horticultural therapy on vulnerability and resistance to substance abuse among incarcerated offenders. *Journal of Offender Rehabilitation, 29*(3/4), 183-193.

Ryff, C. D., & Keyes, C. L. (1995). The structure of psychological well-being revisited. *Journal of Personality and Social Psychology, 69*(4), 719–727.

Sieradzki, S. (2006). Documentation: The professional process of recording outcomes. In R. L. Haller & C. L. Kramer (Eds.), *Horticultural therapy methods: Making connections in health care, human service, and community* programs (pp. 87-104). Binghamton, NY: Haworth Press.

Sheikh, J. I., & Yesavage, J. A. (1986). Geriatric Depression Scale (GDS): Recent evidence and development of a shorter version. *Clinical Gerontologist, 5*(1/2), 165-173.

Ulrich, R. S. (2000). Effects of health facility interior design on well-being: Theory and scientific research. *Journal of Health Care Design, 3,* 97-109.

Ulrich, R. S., & Parsons, R. (1992). Influences on passive experiences with plants on individual well-being and health. In D. Relf (Ed.), *The role of horticulture in human well-being and social development* (pp. 93-105). Portland, OR: Timber Press.

U.S. Census Bureau. (2013). *2012 national population projections.* Retrieved from www.census.gov/population/projections/data/national/2012.html.

Wang, D., & MacMillan, T. (2013). The benefits of gardening for older adults: A systematic review of the literature. *Activities, Adaptation, and Aging, 37*(2),153-181.

Chapter 11: Building Objects for Identity and Biography

Priscilla Dunk-West

Introduction

Found and repurposed objects can offer unique opportunities for self-expression given that the meaning attached to commonly found items can be re-worked to create a symbolic self or be used to form an emotional state. In this chapter, the use of objects in social work and the helping professions are explored. In particular, the focus of this chapter is to understand how objects can help to symbolise identity and the self in relation to others. The work of George Herbert Mead underpins the approach to identity taken in this chapter who suggests that the self is produced through social interaction. Thus objects are both a literal externalisation of identity as well as a metaphor for the self. The use of objects in one-to-one work with clients or small group dialogue is discussed and the range of potential uses for objects in the helping professions are reviewed. A case is made for how these objects can be used make meaning, which is particularly relevant to work related to identity. This chapter begins with an exploration of how visual representations can help us to make sense of who we are and our place is in the social world. Secondly, the use of objects and Lego are considered in practice and research. In particular, I offer an account of the use of both of these in my practice as a counsellor and later as a researcher. The chapter concludes by providing some benefits and potential challenges in the use of objects and Lego in working with others to discover new expressions of identity, biography, and the external world and tips for practitioners when undertaking identity work with objects.

To offer another perspective on the use of repurposed objects in practice, Caron Leader discusses the use of sand tray therapy. As a therapist, she seeks to incorporate creativity into her work with clients, and sand tray allows client to create a representation of their world through the use of toys, photographs, household objects, and of course, the sand.

The Rise of Visual Identities

In contemporary society, visual representations of identity are plentiful. Social media relies upon the visual interaction between an individual or group and a broader audience. Similarly, social media sites require the user to represent themselves and to develop and maintain an identity which is represented through text and images. This "newer" way of creating identity is one of the features of our modern world in which technological change and uncertainty co-exist alongside an increased "reflexive" engagement with the self (Giddens, 1991).

Reflexivity involves acting as a result of a reflection. It involves an ongoing change in behaviour as a direct result of thinking about the past, and a desire to be "better" is part of this mindset. However, we do not all reflect equally (Skeggs, 1997, 2004). The idea that we are constantly aware of our own identity—and constantly update and alter the identity that we project into the world— requires individuals to have self-awareness in relation to others. This demands that individuals equally have the capacity, resources, time, and opportunity to reflect and the ability to change their circumstances. Things like class, culture, and gender impact upon one's ability to reflexively engage (Skeggs, 2004), which means that although individuals may engage in technologies in which identity is represented visually, they may not always understand how it is representative of a fragmentation in traditional communication.

However, it is important to acknowledge that the ways in which we communicate (e.g., ideas about ourselves in relation to others) is changing, and this can be a good thing. The traditional model of therapy is for a client to sit with a professional and talk about her/himself. The "problem" is assumed to reside within the individual in her/his psyche or internal world of the mind (Reiff, 1966). However, sociologist George Herbert Mead offers an alternative theory of self; that is, the mind is merely a concept, which is created through social interaction (Mead 1913, 1934). This theory underscores the importance of the people around us and the context where social interaction occurs.

The ways in which we present ourselves to others may be seen as a kind of performance (Goffman, 1959). The way we behave, our gestures, tone of voice, and how we dress are all examples of ways that we can communicate to others. We "read" the identities of others through these overt and very subtle narratives that others tell through their movements, voice, what they say, how they say it, how they interact with their environment, and so on. This perspective reminds us to be critical of the view that personality is something that is fixed and real. Rather than merely understanding the world through the study of individuals, a focus on the role of society is an important aspect to understanding identity. The connection between the personal and the social is explored in this chapter, though this is a big undertaking. Specifically, the focus is on "external" identity, and the way it can be explored through objects. Who we are depends upon our contexts and biographies, and in contemporary life, we visually project our identities.

There are various examples to demonstrate the growth of visual methods to represent identity. Refrigerator doors, pin/bulletin boards, and other spaces in which photographs, objects, or notes are put together in a kind of collage are used to communicate to others important information about its creator (Gauntlett, 2007). These sorts of visual representations of identity also tell us about society and the importance society places on images. The meaning of an image or an object depends on who has the object and what it means to both society and themselves. For example, a recent study explored footwear and identity, which has meaning beyond its utilitarian uses in contemporary society (Hockey, Dilley, Robinson, & Sherlock, 2013). The authors note that:

> Shoes are...being ascribed the capacity to transcend the functional and even the fashionable–to have implications for identity itself. Through the skills of designers and advertisers, they are seen to achieve symbolic efficacy and transformative, even magical powers (Hockey et al., 2013, p. 1).

This study found that shoes connected their owners to key points in their personal biographies; therefore, shoes were linked with memories. It is important to understand the connections between individual memory and the object, and the ways in which the same item may hold differing significance for the individual. The connection between the object and one's biography and memory is offered in Whincup's (2004) examples:

> ...in the form of photographs of objects, with their owner's explanations of their meaning–show how people imbue everyday objects with special meanings. A cheap toy or an empty champagne bottle, for example, can have massive amounts of sentimental meaning to one individual, because of the personal stories and memories they are associated with, even though the items would be worthless to anyone else (as cited in Gauntlett, 2007, p. 140).

People continue to make new connections with novel objects, and visual methods offer a way to interpret and represent ourselves in our social world. These other forms of communication enable people to reflect, interact physically with an object or objects and to form new understandings. A recent study helps illustrate the meaning-making that can occur, in this case when an object is found and then repurposed. Camic (2010) surveyed individuals who made use of found objects in order to study their utilisation of them. Results suggest that these found objects were creatively used, and Camic (2010) posits that, "the interaction between finder and object is an attempt to make meaning of an object that has been found" (p. 89).

Case Example: How are Objects Used in Research?

The use of Lego to represent identity was developed by sociologist David Gauntlett (2007) who developed a variation of "Lego serious play."

> Lego Serious Play enhances participants' insight, commitments and confidence by engaging them in a hands-on, minds-on experience. Worldwide, companies on five continents have used Lego Serious Play applications to improve strategic planning, manage successful projects and build better teams. In practical terms, Lego Serious Play is a concept and methodology that helps organisations have more effective meetings

> to solve complex strategic issues (Lego Serious Play marketing material, 2006 as cited in Gauntlett, 2007, p. 129).

The physical manipulation inherent to Lego creates a prolonged interaction because the participant needs to think about and construct her/his object. Adapting Gauntlett's (2007) methodological approach to identity with Lego, I had participants build metaphorical models of their identities. Specifically, final year social work students were asked to build a model of their social work self/identity. Preliminary findings suggest that the use of Lego is helping participants to frame a story that is difficult to articulate; one that might not otherwise be evident if we relied on dialogue only.

In the photograph *Lego Model of Identity*, the participant, Leanne (a pseudonym), has constructed a scene involving two areas. The area to the right of the image depicts the social worker on the telephone, seated. The client is depicted as the figure approaching the desk. There is a doorway between this office environment and the other space (on the left of the image). The doorway is an opening, but does not contain a door. Leanne reported that the four blocks above the doorway represented the movement between the "home" and "work" identities. The home identity to the left of the picture shows a cat, some pizzas, flowers, and a tree. There is also a truck parked outside. Leanne said, "The car, I guess, represents the outreach nature of the job and the way that you have to go out there. You can't just sit in one spot and expect clients to come to you." She went on to describe her model:

> ... sometimes as a social worker I feel like I'm sort of between different worlds. This is my client's world. They do put walls up. But sometimes we see through a little window into their life. So that's that representation. I haven't put a roof on there because I feel like sometimes they don't have that protection that we have. This is me. And she wouldn't sit on her chair properly because of her hair. But I thought it's interesting I can put her on the edge of her seat, because sometimes I do feel like I'm on the edge of my seat like, "What's going to happen next?" and the crisis and the chaos.

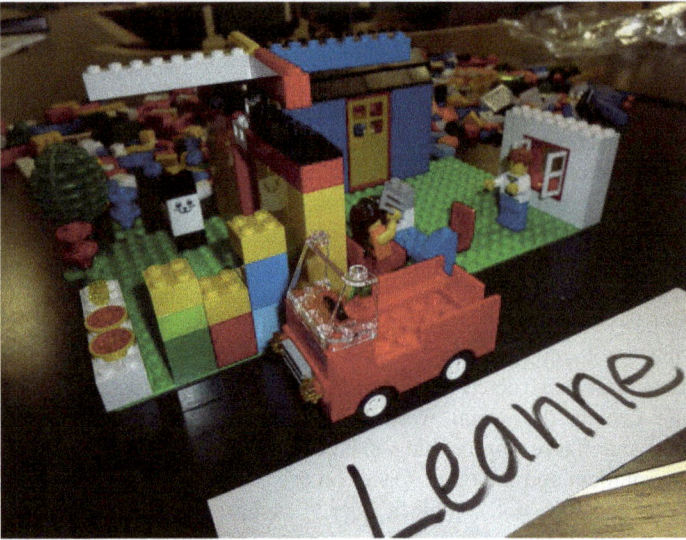

Title: *Lego Model of Identity.*

There is a clear connection between both the possibilities and limits to working with this kind of medium. Unlike other materials, such as modelling clay or paint, there are some limitations in the ways in which the blocks and pieces of Lego can be constructed, since they lock into place with one another. Leanne spoke of the inability to fit the figure onto the chair properly (because of the hair on the figure), and she accommodated for this in her explanation about being "on the edge" of one's seat as being an anticipatory aspect to social work where there is a requirement for spontaneity.

In this kind of research, participants used real-world, everyday objects to represent both biographically relevant, but also socially "readable" items. This resonates with Gauntlett's (2007) research in which

> ...some ideas were represented in mostly very similar ways. For example, people were very frequently used to represent *family*. A spirit of *openness* was represented by open doors, windows and transparent pieces. Participants often built houses to represent the importance of their home life (italics added for emphasis; p. 156).

One of the reasons that research with Lego appeals to me, as someone who has incorporated Mead's work into my theorising about social work identity (Dunk-West, 2013), is that Mead argues that childhood is an important time for children to learn through play and games (Mead, 1913). Through using a resource which is associated with children's play, my hope was to create an environment which allows for people to move beyond traditional ways of communicating. Identity is a somewhat difficult concept for people to articulate, but Lego can help depict self-reflection. It also helps increase understanding about the ways in which we *interact* with the world around us. This idea—that the self is produced through social interaction—is core to Mead's scholarship (Mead, 1913, 1925, 1929).

Objects and the Helping Professions

Emphasising the external has many benefits. In a literal sense, the use of objects physically produces a representation of who we are, and figuratively, objects offer an alternative way to focus on the internal mind of the individual. For example, many therapeutic approaches (e.g., narrative therapy) argue that practitioners ought to "externalise" problems so that they can be seen as separate from the individual. Separating the individual from the problem helps the client to better understand her/himself as well as society and come to realize that s/he is not the "problem." Externalising people's stories or narratives can also help them to objectively understand the contextual factors which influence our experiences in day-to-day life (White & Epston, 1990; Morgan, 2000). Making these connections—that is, the personal with the societal—can bring about a richness for the helping relationship as a new communicative activity is created. The use of objects external to individuals can be helpful to this endeavour.

It is important to gain some clarity about what constitutes an object. Objects can be understood as anything external to the individual. As we have seen, shoes are external to the individual, yet they are rich with meaning and retain personal as well as social significance. The same may be said for found objects. For the purposes of the helping relationship, it is preferable to use objects that do not belong to the individual or groups with whom we are working. These objects may be thought of as "repurposed" since they are being used in a new way. Items that can be combined to form a story or a map are useful in the articulation of a particular narrative, and as such, it is best if objects are small enough to handle easily. Here are a few examples of repurposed objects that can be used in the helping professions to work with clients:

- A small ball
- A small piece of string
- Small children's toys, such as toy ducks, soldiers, animals, or toys that move (e.g., jack-in-the-box, puzzle, blocks, wind up toys)
- A paperweight
- Screws, nails, and nuts
- A blindfold
- A watch or other jewellery
- A small plant, such as a cactus

Arts are often underappreciated in the everyday work of helping professionals (Dillenburger, 1992). Yet, the role of the arts in practical settings has been carefully documented and embedded into work with particular groups including university students (Rose, 1996, 2012) and children (Landreth, 2012). This work has been contexualised as an activity that relies on the imagination of others to shed light onto a particular situation. As such, the client sits opposite the helper and is expected to talk about what has brought her/him to seek out help. The imagination is often required because such conversations expect the client to describe their past and present and imagine their future. Therapy generally involves a dialogue that leads the client to gain to insight about her/himself; something they would not have already had. As discussed earlier, this kind of therapy assumes an identity, which is internal, idiosyncratic, and individualised. Although objects and artwork can be used to help clients resolve emotional conflict or trauma, the use of objects in understanding and communicating identity is examined in this portion of the chapter (Note: Other therapeutic uses of repurposed objects can be found at the end of the chapter in the section entitled *Sand Tray Play: Creating One's Internal World through the Use of Repurposed Objects.*)

Exploring identity leads to questions about social expectations associated with age, gender, class, sexual identity, and other aspects of difference. These kinds of explorations can help individuals to understand their lived experiences in the context of social expectations. Whereas therapy might involve understanding the hidden or unconscious thoughts, which influence behaviour, examining identity has more of an outward facing focus. Sociological social work encourages practitioners to look at the world around them (Dunk-West & Verity, 2013). Similarly, identity work encourages the participant to understand the taken for granted, everyday assumptions and social norms which shape society's expectations of them (Lefebvre, 1991).

This focus on "identity" or "self" can help individuals understand themselves in relationship to society. Identity is a difficult concept to describe and convey, but objects can help make sense of how identity is played out in people's lives. For example, the role of the visual is found in the ways that we engage with popular culture such as through film watching (Monaco, 1981) or visual arts (Berger, 1977). It has impacted the way that we communicate as well. "Emoticons" may represent our need to imbue greater meaning and emotion to our words, which may signify a shift towards an increasingly visual culture.

It is widely accepted that humans communicate many nuances of identity through social interaction. Gestures, eye contact, body position, and verbal communication are all conduits through which meaning is conveyed and received. Although these are part of day-to-day life, they are often underappreciated and unnoticed. Take a moment, for example, to consider how one person can communicate to another that they are angry. The furrowing of the brows or grimace can serve to illustrate one's mood, whether intentionally or unintentionally. There is considerable evidence that a range of factors affect the ways in which we communicate—our culture, class, age, and gender for example. Practitioners who are adept at working with different groups of people will often talk about the importance of helping professionals being able to *respond* to differing communicative styles. This involves a reflexive understanding of how one comes across and the skills in using different gestures, language, styles, and actions depending on the context (Cournoyer, 2010). Developing effective communicative skills requires understanding the individual(s) with whom one works. Yet there is no guarantee that what might work with one person will work with another client. For example, communicating with a young person might involve talking about music, artwork, body modification, and other forms of self-expression. Each of these might be symbolic to a particular person for a range of reasons. Similarly, communicating with a couple in a counselling context might involve talking, laughing, and joking. It might also involve the use of diagrams and humour.

Case Example: How are Objects Used in Practice?

In the context of my counselling work, I began using external tools to help with communication. Inspired initially by narrative therapy and the role of identity in meaning-making, I began collecting little objects that could be used in the counselling room. All of the objects were purchased for the sole purpose of facilitating communication with my clients. I did not use objects of my own given the symbolic and biographical attachments we can have to particular objects (Hockey et al., 2013) and hoped to avoid projecting my meanings of objects into the interaction with my clients.

Twirling Girl Toy Figure (depicted in the photograph below) is a child's wooden toy and an example of an object that can be used to symbolise how someone is feeling in relation to the world around her/him. The object can be turned, which pushes the wooden person over the bar. One can imagine a client saying "I am forever jumping around and around for those around me... I find it hard to slow down" or "I chose this object because it shows someone on top of the world!" or "Day after day I do the same thing!" These are just some possibilities of what could be endless ways in which a person might describe how they see themselves and what the object might symbolise for them at one particular moment in time. Who we are emerges through the exchanges we have with other people; in order for me to talk to my friend, a sense of *who I am* is present. In this way the self is constituted and re-constituted, dependent on social interaction, physical location, and context. When we think about identity in this way, as contingent and changing, dynamic and ethereal, words can fail to depict such a complex and shifting terrain. Objects can assist in providing a metaphorical account of identity; a contextual and "still" form which balances the increasingly fragmented and shifting life in contemporary society.

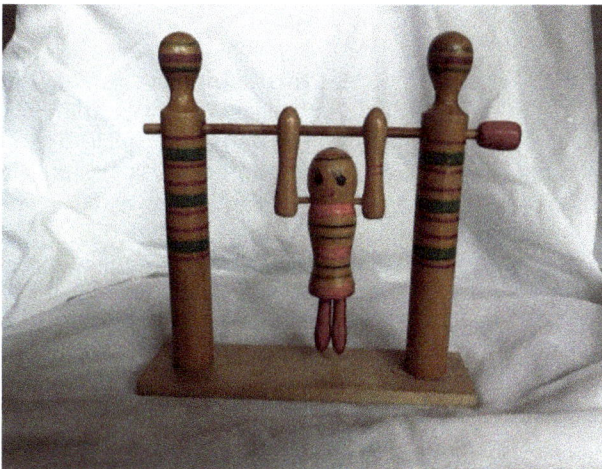

Title: *Twirling Girl Toy Figure.*

Benefits and Potential Challenges

The use of objects and Lego offers new ways to communicate and bring new meaning to understanding both identity and one's place in the social world. Unlike traditional models of identity in which the internal world is explored through "talk therapies," the symbolic and literal "external" object speaks of a broader theoretical tradition (Mead, 1913), which highlights the interactive space as creating identities. The meaning that others bring to particular objects is important to finding new meanings for one's identity, which requires new insights. For these reasons, the use of objects and Lego has much to offer the world of practice and research. Practitioners wishing to use these methods simply need the capacity to work with these materials, the sensibility to play, the understanding of the role of play in communication, and the ability to be mindful of how aspects of difference are relevant to selecting the most appropriate method for the people with whom we work.

Although the use of objects and Lego have been argued to promote new ways of relating to the people with whom we work, it is important to recognise the potential limitations to using them. Just as objects can be recognised as being associated with a particular meaning, such as a car with transport, a kitchen with food preparation/consumption, so too can the very materials we work with be coded with particular significance. When used in practice, found objects and Lego need to be understood as cultural artifacts. For example, an adult who played with Lego as a child might be more willing to engage with this medium since they will understand that they can use blocks and other pieces for construction. Although Lego has historically been represented as gender neutral, there has been a recent move to diversify the colours used. For example, it is now possible to purchase pink and blue Lego packs, two colours, which are heavily associated with girls and boys respectively. For the practitioner thinking about using Lego, these considerations must be built into the design of the work.

Similarly, found objects must be seen as potentially significant to individuals, but also as socially coded. This means that class, (dis)ability, gender, and other aspects of difference will bring new meanings to the object. Objects also have an historical context embedded into their meaning. The material from which a child's toy is made, for example, will tell us something about not only where the item might be made, but also when and how it was made. Let us take one example of a marker of difference, in this case, age. Since it is through the process of socialisation that children learn about the meanings attached to certain symbols and objects (Mead, 1913), the age at which a child comes to an object will impact their reading of that object. If a child takes an object—say a drink coaster—it might be used as a telephone, a baby, or a hat. This is a very unidirectional reading of an object, and children's play can be much more complex because they do not think in this "rational" manner (Piaget, 1964, 1973). Because children are not limited to adult style cognition and reasoning (Vygotsky, 1962), using an object to communicate differently has the potential to limit creative expression as opposed to freeing it up. This is not to say that objects are not appropriate to use when communicating with children; it is merely important for the person working with the child to recognise that they may need to suspend their way of understanding objects in order to understand the ways in which children experience and make sense of the world around them. There is still some evidence that the ways in which children play are dictated by socially prescribed roles for men and women; that is, childhood play replicates gender divisions in society (Lever, 1978).

There is a myriad of other considerations, which bear thinking through in terms of identity work and the use of objects. For the practitioner wishing to use objects and/or Lego in their work, the following questions can assist in providing a tool to evaluate the usefulness of this kind of communicative device to their work:

- What is it that I want to find out?
- What are the potential benefits to using this approach with my clients?
- How does gender relate to the use of objects/Lego? For example, will boys/men find it easier to relate to this kind of communication?
- Are the objects/Lego tasks age-specific? Why?
- What is the connection between my practice approach and the use of objects/Lego?
- Are the participants going to be able to physically use the materials?
- How will I use the activity? Will I follow up with questions or conversations after the activity is completed? Or will we speak as we go?
- Is it appropriate to record my interactions and the products of the session? What ethics approval processes do I need in my organisational context?
- How will I evaluate the use of these methods?

By examining these questions within the context of practice/research, the practitioner will be better prepared for overcoming obstacles as they occur during the process. Much like other methods, clients/participants will present with their own perspective on how the interaction should occur.

Ethical Considerations

It is of upmost importance that clients/participants gain something from their work with objects. The ethical principles of nonmalificence and beneficence (Beauchamp & Childress, 1989) are relevant in this context—do not harm and work to do good. The practitioner should start where the individual is. In other words, the practitioner may challenge the participant to stretch, but it is also important that to limit the work to what the client thinks is best.

Similarly, as with any work with individuals, it is imperative to work in partnership. This means gaining consent from clients/participants prior to their engagement in identity exploration using objects. An explanation of how the objects may be used, the practitioner's role in the process, and the goal of the activity is a good place to start. Clients/participants may feel uncomfortable or unsure of themselves as they contemplate using a new, innovative way to communicate. Reassurance that there is no "wrong way" to proceed may help allay their fears or anxieties about the process.

Tips for Practitioners

1. **Be clear that the focus of this work is to examine social expectations of individuals**. Whereas therapeutic work might draw from ideas of subjectivity, using objects to understand identity draws from sociological perspectives. This means that the practitioner needs to draw out the significance of social expectations placed upon individuals, understand the process of socialisation, and help the participant to connect these ideas to their own experiences and biographies.

2. **If clients are "doing it wrong," go with it.** There really is no right or wrong way to using objects to help explore identity. Objects can represent themselves, aspects of themselves, others, social institutions, emotions… the list is endless.

3. **Test out which objects are working well with people**. If there are certain types of objects that do not seem to resonate with clients, seek out some additional objects. Be aware of gender and other aspects of difference when selecting objects. Since this is a type of play, there are some objects and toys that are socially coded as male or female.

4. **Rotate the objects being used when consistently working with clients.** This will help reach new insights or conversations.

5. **Display the objects in a prominent place.** People who are curious about the objects can easily have a look at them, handle them, and ask what they are for. Practitioners can describe how they are used and ask if they would like to try working with them either now or in the future.

6. **Limit the amount of the objects to around 20**. It is useful to experiment with the ideal number. You want participants to have choices, but you also do not want them to feel overwhelmed by choice.

7. **Objects used for work with people can, and perhaps should, include children's toys**. Toys can make up some of the collection of objects or consist of the whole collection. As previously discussed, Lego has been used to help people explore their identities. It is worth thinking about toys or games and seeing if they are worth adapting for the purposes of working with people around identity.

8. **In everyday life we interact with a number of objects**. These can be useful to include in the collection of objects. Experiment to see which objects are more meaningful or useful to people. These might include pens, soap, keys, small items of jewellery or clothing, cups, and so on.

9. **Experiment with silence.** This will help you determine if it is better to be silent while the client/participant constructs their model. The alternative is to talk to the participant while they are making their collage or mapping out their creation. The practitioner can also set the task. For example, you could ask the participant/client to make a collage of how s/he sees her/himself right now and leave the room. This can allow the participant to feel more freedom to "get it wrong" or think without having the pressure to complete the task with an audience.

10. **Have fun!** Practitioners and the people with whom they work are using an alternative to conversation. This can be confronting to clients/participants so acknowledging that this kind of work can feel a bit strange can help to normalise feelings of ill ease. Practitioners ought to

encourage a playfulness, which enables the people with whom they work to open up new channels for communication and meaning.

Recommended Readings and Resources

Gauntlett, D. (2007). *Creative explorations: New approaches to identities and audiences*. London: Routledge.

Rose, G. (2012). *Visual methodologies: An introduction to interpreting visual materials* (3rd ed.). London: Sage.

References

Beauchamp, T. L., & Childress, J. F. (1989). *Principles of biomedical ethics*. New York: Oxford University Press.

Berger, J. (1977). *Ways of seeing*. London: Penguin Books.

Camic, P. M. (2010). From trashed to treasured: A grounded theory analysis of the found object. *Psychology of Aesthetics, Creativity, and the Arts, 4*(2), 81-92.

Cournoyer, B. (2010). *The social work skills workbook*. Belmont, CA: Brooks Cole.

Dillenburger, K. (1992). Communicating with children: The use of art in social work. *Practice, 6*(2), 126-134.

Dunk-West, P. (2013). *How to be a social worker: A critical guide for students*. Basingstoke, UK: Palgrave Macmillan.

Dunk-West, P., & Verity, F. (2013). *Sociological social work*. Surrey, UK: Ashgate.

Gauntlett, D. (2007). *Creative explorations: New approaches to identities and audiences*. London: Routledge.

Giddens, A. (1991). *Modernity and self-identity: Self and society in the late modern age*. Cambridge: Polity.

Goffman, E. (1959). *The presentation of self in everyday life*. New York: Anchor Books.

Hockey, J., Dilley, R., Robinson, V., & Sherlock, A. (2013). Worn shoes: Identity, memory and footwear. *Sociological Research Online, 18*(1), 20.

Landreth, G. (2012). *Play therapy: The art of the relationship*. New York: Routledge.

Lefebvre, H. (1991). *Critique of everyday life: Introduction* (Vol. 1). London: Verso.

Lever, J. (1978). Sex differences in the complexity of children's play and games. *American Sociological Review, 43(*4), 471-483.

Mead, G. H. (1913). The social self. In F. C. Silva (Ed.), *G.H. Mead: A reader*. Abingdon, UK: Routledge.

Mead, G. H. (1925). The genesis of the self and social control. In F. C. Silva (Ed.), *G.H. Mead: A reader*. Abingdon, UK: Routledge.

Mead, G. H. (1929). The nature of the past. In F. C. Silva (Ed.), *G.H. Mead: A reader*. Abingdon, UK: Routledge.

Mead, G. H. (1934). *Mind, self and society from the standpoint of a social behaviourist*. Chicago, IL: Chicago University Press.

Monaco, J. (1981). *How to read a film: The art, technology, lanuage, history, and theory of film and media.* Oxford: Oxford University Press.

Morgan, A. (2000). *What is narrative therapy? An easy-to-read introduction.* Adelaide South Australia: Dulwich Centre Publications.

Piaget, J. (1964). *The early growth of logic in the child.* London: Routledge.

Piaget, J. (1973). *The child's conception of the world.* London: Paladin.

Reiff, P. (1966). *The triumph of the therapeutic: Uses of faith after Freud.* New York: Harper & Row.

Rose, G. (1996). Teaching visualised geographies: Towards a methodology for the interpretation of visual materials. *Journal of Geography in Higher Education, 20*(3), 281-294.

Rose, G. (2012). *Visual methodologies: An introduction to interpreting visual materials.* London: Sage.

Skeggs, B. (1997). *Formations of class and gender: Becoming respectable.* London: Sage.

Skeggs, B. (2004). *Class, self, culture.* London: Routledge.

Vygotsky, L. S. (1962). *Thought and language.* Cambridge: M.I.T. Press.

White, M., & Epston, D. (1990). *Narrative means to therapeutic ends.* New York: Norton.

Sand Tray Play: Creating One's Internal World through the Use of Repurposed Objects

Caron Leader

Sand tray play is a form of expressive therapy that allows clients to express their emotional and cognitive processes through play in sand. This expressive play symbolically represents the individual's life experiences and provides the opportunity for unconscious processes to become manifest through an unfolding therapeutic experience (De Domenico, 1999). Sand tray play was developed in the 1920s (initially called the Method World Pictures) by Margaret Lowenfeld and can be described as non-directed, free, and spontaneous play. Deemed therapeutic for children, adults, families, and couples, sand try play can be used across the lifespan and is appropriate for a range of different psychological issues (De Domenico, 1995). The decision to introduce sand play is based on a difficulty with verbal expression, therapeutic trust, timing, and the client's willingness to try the approach.

First, a client is introduced to sand tray therapy by allowing her/him to get acquainted with the sand. They can touch the sand, move it, get the sand wet, and/or build their own world in the sand. The trays measure roughly two-feet-by-two-feet and are three-feet deep, and the sand is filled about halfway in the tray. The tray is placed on a waist-high table and the play begins. Creations may be enhanced with the addition of miniature images or other repurposed items—toys, emblems from games, or household objects. The builder of the world chooses whatever draws or repels them, and items are used to depict any aspect of life, including elements of nature, animals, fictional characters, and vehicles amongst others. Construction and art materials such as paper, tape, ribbon, fabric, and wood can be added to enhance the building process or photographs can be used to add further dimension to the world. In the photograph below, the sand tray area in my office is shown. What emerges is a world in the limited space of the sand tray that reflects aspects of the builder's life experience in a very real, concentrated, and illuminating manner. The building process itself may be completed in one session or it could require several sessions. Photographs are used to chronicle the world for the builder, which are then used later for further reflection or for future reference. The photograph, *Caron's Sand Tray*, illustrates a created scene.

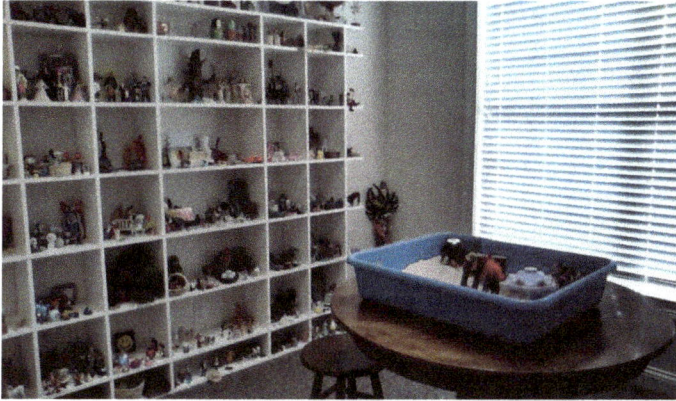

Title: *Sand Tray Area.*
Photo by: Caron Leader.

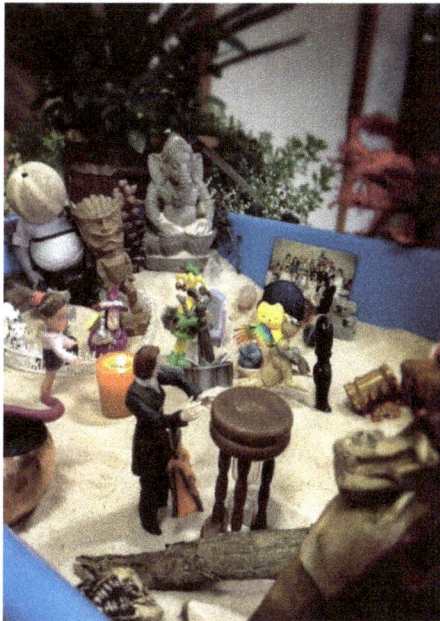

Title: *Caron's Sand Tray.*
Photo by: Caron Leader.

The theoretical premise for this process is that there is a "builder" of this sand tray world and a "witness" to the building process and product. The practitioner stands by observing and experiencing the creation of this new world as the builder adds elements and arranges or re-arranges the composition. During this free and spontaneous play, the builder is in charge of the world, and the practitioner is the silent but attentive witness. Through the silent, here and now experience, the practitioner is granted access into the builder's internal reality. Being present in the moment is critical for establishing safety that supports the builder's unconscious process to emerge into consciousness. The practitioner's skill at reflection becomes key here. Matching movements, breathing, and pace provides subtle encouragement for the builder to enter the psyche. Once the world is complete, a shared experiencing of the sand tray is initiated, which further enriches the builder's experience. As the world is shared, the practitioner asks specific questions about the newly created world— not regarding the process of building, but rather about the world and the images themselves. These probing questions urge the builder to process their creation on a much deeper level, and something powerful happens in this therapeutic process as the practitioner joins with the builder and actually experiences her/his world. Builders are encouraged to freely express themselves in order to achieve their personal goals, and this shared experience acts to further integrate the changes that occur during the process of building (De Domenico, 1999).

Directed sand play experiences can also be used therapeutically (De Domenico, 1995). These techniques rely on more specific instructions and interactions between the practitioner and the builder. For example, the therapist might ask the builder to reenact a particular experience, such as a nightmare or accident (e.g., car, sports, etc.), to further discover key elements of this experience and create greater understanding of the builder's perspective. Alternatively, the sand tray can be used as a didactic exercise. The therapist might use images to depict feeling states and ask the builder to role-play by interacting with the images. This type of interaction can produce a quicker and deeper learning of a desired positive behavior. For example, a child might be inappropriately expressing anger. The sand play can be arranged to visually depict positive expression of anger. Another directed sand play technique involves pairing two opposite types of images and asking the builder to use these in creating their world (e.g., lion and lamb; De Domenico, 1995). Many free and directed play techniques are possible; this approach to practice is only limited by the practitioner's imagination.

In sum, this type of expressive therapy can be helpful when talk therapy is not enough; words alone do not always suffice in the communication of human experience. Clients who create scenes and worlds through sand tray therapy are forced to think differently, often times using the sand to portray experiences and emotions that words may only hint at. An experiential tool that can be readily adapted to individuals, couples, and groups is therapeutically valuable. It is a creative vehicle that can produce dramatic results and provide another medium for communication and expression.

Recommended Readings and Resources

Association for Play Therapy. (2014). Resources and trainings available at: http://www.a4pt.org/search.cfm?task=results&requesttimeout=1200.

Bowyer, R. (1970). *The Lowenfeld world technique*. Oxford: Pergamon Press.

De Domenico, G. (2000). The phenomenology of seeking, finding and being self. *Sandtray Newtwork Journal*, Winter.

Dundas, E. (1978). *Symbols come alive in the sand*. Berkeley: Author.

Jung, C. G. (1971). *The portable Jung*. J. Campbell (Ed.) New York: Viking.

Jung, C. G. (1963). *Memories, dreams and reflections*. New York: Random House.

Sand play therapists of America. (2014). Resources and trainings available at: www.sandplay.org

Vision quest into symbolic reality. (n.d.) Information and trainings available at: http://vision-quest.us.

References

De Domenico, G. (1999). Experiential dimensions of sandplay: Sandplay-worldplay theory and methods. *Sandtray Network Journal*, Winter.

De Domenico, G. (1995). *Sand tray world play: A comprehensive guide to the use of the sand tray in psychotherapeutic and transformational settings.* Oakland, CA: Vision Quest Images.

Chapter 12: Community Theatre: Approaches, Challenges, and Outcomes

Russell Fewster & Susan Harris

The arts help us to understand ourselves [and] provide us with insights that instil a sense of community and identity (South Australian Department for Education and Child Development, 2010).

Introduction

Art is integral to our daily lives and is vital to a vibrant, healthy community. Community art, notably theatre, is accessible and is not impeded by high ticket/admission prices to view it. Community theatre can refer to a self-appointed, self-determining group of people creating theatre for a common purpose; professional artists collaborating with a community; or theatre which is created on behalf of a culturally disadvantaged community. In all instances, community consultation and dialogue is crucial to the creative process. Culturally, a community, like any other organisation, is constructed and developed by its members who contribute to the group their own individual sets of life experiences, personal ethos, belief system, and perspective. Community theatre is not just about imparting or communicating messages; it is about the *act* of communication. Theatre affects participants, who in turn, influence each other as well as the art that is being created. If theatre is to serve the needs of a community in the form of an audience, it must seek to ensure those audience members are actively engaged rather than passive observers. An audience engagement increases the likelihood for social activism and change. As such, community theatre has purpose. It can be a vehicle for a community's cultural development, arts enrichment, public awareness, or be a voice for social change.

This chapter is written in two parts: Russell Fewster gives an overview of the philosophical origins of community theatre before considering its impact on newer forms such as verbatim and documentary theatre. Sue Harris then discusses the philosophical and practical challenges for arts practitioners working within communities in the new millennium. This chapter charts the origins and animating aesthetic principles underpinning community theatre practice and how theatre created for specific communities is realised. Two case studies are offered along with ethical considerations and tips for practitioners.

Methods of Practice: Philosophical Inspiration

In tracing the philosophical underpinnings of community theatre, the aesthetic principles and practices of 20th Century German playwright Bertolt Brecht provide a helpful starting point. Brecht's "innovations" give useful ways at looking at the broad intentions of community theatre. The fundamental tenet underlying community theatre is the capacity for change: change in a community's attitudes and actions towards a particular issue or situation. In his "epic theatre," Brecht (1974) outlined change as key to overcoming what he saw as the limitations of "dramatic theatre." This included turning the spectator from an observer into someone who has "capacity for action … take[s] decisions [and] …is alterable and able to alter their "narrative" (as cited in Willet, 1982, p.37). Above all Brecht (1974) saw humans as being part of "a process," and once they are energised, they are capable of intervening and changing the world around them.

The animating current that underlies community theatre is to involve the participants and spectators in a process that invites change. This holds true whether the theatre is created within, with, or for a particular community, and the goal is to empower community members. The focus of the project can increase awareness regarding that community, their needs, and aspirations. Brecht's subject matter with its concern for the "human being as the object of enquiry" manifests in his notion of *Lehrstück* or learning play, a clear inspiration for community theatre. The underlying principle of *Lehrstück* is the idea that "moral and political lessons could best be taught by participation in an actual performance" (Brecht as cited in Willet, 1982, p. 33).

We would extend this sense of "participation" to both performer and spectator as ownership and identity formation are inextricably linked to the collaboration between artists and community. This search for identity is as much for artists working within a specific community as for the community themselves. Both popular and increasingly sophisticated theatre forms have developed out of the community immersion of professional artists. This is closely linked to the notion of the "learning play" and the forerunner of theatre in education companies in the United Kingdom and Australia and grassroots theatre companies in the United States that immerse themselves in communities to develop a company-wide participation in community collaboration. This artist-in-residence approach was later formalised by funding and practices in community theatre.

Community Theatre: Formalisation and Transformation

If theatre has traditionally been entwined with communities as a means of expression of community issues, stories, and moral fables, then it has gained increasing contemporary currency. Slowly, the white male Anglo presence on stage and screen has been replaced with women and people of diverse backgrounds, which reflects the multicultural community world where we live.

One of the goals of community theatre is to tell the stories of those outside the "mainstream" narrative, and it continues to be successful in this effort.

The term "applied theatre" has recently emerged and includes a number of community theatre practices such as: "grassroots theatre, social theatre, political theatre, and radical theatre" (Prendergast & Saxton, 2009, p.6-7). The notion of "applied theatre" frequently refers to the application of theatre practices in non-traditional settings such as prisons, schools, or other locations that are important to the community (Prentki & Preston, 2009). Moreover, this application has increasingly extended to non-Western countries and communities. In this way, theatre has broadened its connection to society by involvement in communities previously untouched by theatrical forms and approaches. Some key examples of this metamorphosis are illustrated through the infusion of community theatre into new forms of production such as refugee theatre and documentary theatre.

Refugee Theatre

Community theatre can be defined as content-specific theatre that emerges within the context of a particular community group, which refers to any group that shares a common experience. At times, groups vary in their self-determined status due to the given circumstances of their time. For example, refugees are united by common experiences that are outside of their control, while others debate over whether they "choose" to be refugees or not. As such, this particular community is politicised, and any theatre emerging about this group needs to be viewed within this context.

Refugee theatre is particularly pertinent as the Western world struggles to deal with the increased global movement of asylum seekers. In Australia for example, between 1999 and 2005, there were 30 productions on this theme; however, much of theatre was actually "that of activists and supporters, rather than the refugees themselves" (McCallum, 2006, p. 136). Thus, the refugees were voiceless as they were detained for lengthy periods with limited access to the media. In this instance, theatre is made *about* a particular group by those outside of the experience due to the disempowerment of that group of people. The need for such theatre is diverse in terms of providing an outlet for a human experience that goes untold in mainstream media. Furthermore, this type of theatre can facilitate an in-depth exploration of personal stories, events, and reactions that above all seek to humanise the hidden voices of refugees. In Australia, the telling of biographical stories such as in refugee theatre has blossomed over the last 20 years in the form of documentary theatre, which is known in the United Kingdom and Australia as verbatim theatre and in the United States as testimonial theatre.

Documentary Theatre: Political Perspective[4]

Government censorship may have ensured that very little was seen of asylum seekers by the media; however, theatre may have been in a "good position to tell refugee stories" in the absence of in-depth media documentation (McCallum,

---

[4] This section draws from the PhD dissertation: *An Examination of the Relationship between the Live Performer and Projected Media in Stage Performance* by Russell Fewster, University of Melbourne 2010.

2006, p. 136). Thus, theatre made visible what "border politics"[2] had made invisible. This type of theatre is simultaneously documentary and overtly political and has become known as "verbatim theatre"—the use of the actual text that were spoken by a contemporary public figure, which is then staged in a theatrical setting.

One important example is *The Colour of Justice* (1999) by the United Kingdom–based Tricycle Theatre, who restaged a court hearing. This production demonstrated that the police were incompetent liars who were subsequently still let off by the court. This performance exposed official injustice in the face of public outrage against the falseness of official reports. What the play achieved was to give an outlet for the public to communally recognise that justice had been obstructed by authority—a cathartic release for separate communities that were united by the injustice of the case (see Reinelt, 2006, p. 69-83).

International verbatim works that have directly critiqued the "War on Terror" such as *Stuff Happens* and *Guantanamo* seemed to have sprung primarily from the United Kingdom and then toured to the United States. According to Bottoms (2006), works in the United States have tended to be either "grotesque satire" or more social documentary in nature.[3] Though in regards to the latter, grassroots theatre companies argue that their work is nonetheless inherently political. In the United States, verbatim theatre has perhaps been problematized by a tighter political and artistic climate. For example, the New York Theatre Workshop's production of the play *My Name is Rachel Corrie*, the story of a 23-year-old pro-Palestinian activist, retold from her emails, letters, and diary entries was postponed after concerns of bias were raised by members of the Jewish community, creating outrage (Martin, 2006). The most pertinent criticism was that the play did not balance conflicting views. If "truth" was to be played out, multiple "truths" needed to be displayed. That is, truth is multi-faceted or that ultimately truth is a construction, that is edited by the theatre maker. Martin (2006) comments that: "Governments 'spin' the facts in order to tell stories. Theatre spins them right back to tell different stories" (p.14).

Documentary theatre can therefore be seen to be simultaneously getting to the "truth" of the matter and presenting its own "spin" depending upon the audience's political views and theatrical awareness. Invariably the theatre makers tend to take up positions counter to the prevailing authorities in order to "set the record straight" (Martin, 2006, p.14). Sophisticated multi-media reflections on community and global issues such as refugees, policing, judiciary, war, and terrorism are underlined by an opposition to the ruling establishment's narrative.

---

[2] Ghassan Hage refers to the need for the "rich nations of the first world" (including Australia) to keep "aggressive, non-democratic border politics […] as invisible as possible" i.e., to protect the illusion of a "loving interior" the "hatred and mistrust" of border politics needs to be kept "at the border" p. 31).

[3] Stephen Bottoms gives as examples of satire: Tim Robbin"s *Embedded* (2003), Adriano Shaplin"s *Pugilist Specialist* (2003), and Sam Shepard"s *The God of Hell* (2004) (2006: 57). While for social documentary type works we cite, *The Laramie Project* (2000), an interview-based exploration of the murder of a gay student in Wyoming, which we discuss later in this chapter.

The impulse within community theatre to tell alternative stories is thus a key component of verbatim theatre.

Documentary Theatre: Social Perspectives

One of the aspects of community theatre not touched on previously is its approach to sensitive issues, such as the impact of violence upon communities. Theatre that utilises this approach offers a cathartic release to traumatised communities through well-researched productions. These works are characterised by extensive community consultation and a focus not on the violence itself, but the causes of those traumatic events and their consequences. In this way, documentary theatre has incorporated community healing as one of its goals, even though these companies do not call their work "community theatre." We discuss two examples of this process in the development of the plays: *The Laramie Project*, by New York-based Tectonic Theatre Company, and *Property of the Clan* (later *Blackrock*) by Freewheels Company in Newcastle, Australia.

The interview as the basis for documentary performance reaches its pinnacle in *The Laramie Project* (2000). Following the 1998 murder of Matthew Sheppard, a young gay man in Laramie, Wyoming, director Moises Kaufman and ten members of his theatre company conducted over 200 interviews with the Laramie community. For Kaufman, if it were a "watershed" moment in history, then it would also become a watershed moment for the company. The actors who conducted the interviews and discovered the art of "listening" to the community then worked up scenes or "moments," which they improvised for Kaufman. The resultant play is one of the most widely performed plays in America and internationally. The company returned ten years later to re-interview and chart change. In the aftermath of the crime, the Matthew Sheppard Foundation and the Sheppard Act have been established as well as a commendation in Congress. The impact has been extraordinary. For Kaufman (as cited in Svich, 2003), "In Laramie, it was cathartic. The community talked to itself, using the medium of theatre" (p. 71). That is to say through the sustained immersion of a committed theatre company in their midst, a community was able to open up a dialogue about themselves in response to a traumatic event.

In a similar vein, *The Property of the Clan* (1992) was developed within a specific community in response to the murder of a young person. The late Australian playwright, Nick Enright (1996) recounts how he was asked to write a play by the director (Brian Joyce) of Newcastle's Freewheels TIE company about the then recent rape and murder of Leigh Leigh at a local beach party. Enright initially rejected this as a subject, until he realized that the community was still grieving and needed an outlet to express it. The concern was not the criminal act itself, but rather to "develop the play out of a fatal party, its participants, and its aftermath" (Enright, 1996, p.vii). Much like *The Laramie Project*, the theatre maker's focus was to attempt to shed some understanding on why such violence occurs and its consequences. The play was subsequently reworked as *Blackrock* (1995) by the Sydney Theatre Company and has become one of the most widely performed plays within secondary schools in Australia.

In both works, the theatre makers acted to culturally intervene within a particular community in the aftermath of a violent act utlizing "community theatre as radical cultural intervention" (Kershaw, 1992, p. 13). Theatre provided an alternative means to talking about an issue that had polarised a community when voices within that community had stopped talking due to media intrusion. This method of an interview-based play functioned to reveal those hidden voices. As a pioneer in the field in Australia, Peel (as cited in Capelin, 1995) comments when working within communities of differing viewpoints:

> You're better to get them talking about their situation and find ways of directing them so that they make their own conclusions…you don't change people by…telling them you've got all the answers, you just don't (p. 19).

Theatre-making in this sense is about construction of the interview and the play's dramaturgy; that is, how much of the interview will you include and where will you place it in the play's structure? Peel's (as cited in Capelin, 1995) assertions on approaches to artists working in communities also ring true:

> Firstly, never go where you are uninvited (although this may entail fomenting an invitation); secondly never do one project when you can do three; and thirdly, always ensure you leave something behind (p. 24).

Both works responded to a community's needs, but were interventions rather than direct invitations from the community itself. Both works also resulted in two plays and ongoing contact with the relevant communities. It can be argued that they have indeed also left "something behind"—offering communities an alternative means to self-understanding.

Case Example: *Perish the Thought*

Playwright: Susan Harris; Director: Russell Fewster

Perish the Thought, an issue-based theatre piece, is an adaptation of Harris's book, *A Special Place: Caring for a Parent with Alzheimer's—The Journey,* which was conceived and developed as a voice for the carers' community. Carers are a dispersed community with limited resources for communication between its members. In Australia, the carer-community is significant:

- Almost 2.7 million people in Australia are carers;
- 770,000 people are primary carers; and
- 70% of carers are female (Australian Bureau of Statistics, 2012).

Primary care givers of people with dementia may experience feelings of guilt, isolation, frustration, and helplessness and are sometimes referred to as "the hidden victims of dementia." They are generally isolated due to their circumstances, sometimes even within their own families, and do not often have the opportunity, energy, or strategies in place for social interaction with other carers. This community of carers needs a voice for social change; however, due to fragmentation and isolation, change is difficult.

More than building a body of knowledge about the group and its challenges, *Perish the Thought* sought to connect with the community on all levels: physically, intellectually, and emotionally. So in order to honestly represent this community, facilitators were needed from that community. The playwright had been a primary care-giver for several years as well as a facilitator for creative arts sessions for people with dementia and their carers. Some crew members had had first-hand experience with family members with dementia, and any ensemble member without that personal knowledge was willing to learn. Furthermore, consultation with the peak advocacy body for dementia was also essential as an on-going process.

Issue-based shows demand attention to the audience-actor relationship, which is often pre-determined by the theatre architecture. The play was written with the physical space of the theatre in mind (i.e., audience has tiered seating looking down and into to the stage) to allow for a close relationship to occur between the audience and actors. The topic is intimate; therefore the physical space needed to replicate that intimacy. An audience member's comment to us after a performance, "I wasn't just watching; I was actually there in the room with them," confirmed this sense of intimacy.

Issue-based shows also raise the issue of how to balance truth and art. Do I sacrifice truth for art, or art for truth? Neither must be compromised, but writers and directors need to be creative in their problem solving approach. The play had to be good art to be an effective voice for carers, and for this to occur, the community needed to be moved by the production, feel empathy for the central characters, and derive a sense ownership of the project. This was proven successful through written and verbal feedback and the number of audience members remaining after each performance wanting to share their often unvoiced stories. The show had now become not only a voice for carers but also a catalyst for the carers' voice.

Benefits and Potential Challenges

The use of theatre offers many benefits to practice including its versatility in methods and goals. It may take the form of documentary theatre, drama therapy, or community theatre and cover a wide range of interpersonal/community issues such as violence, gambling, dementia, mental health, trauma, and refugees, just to name a few. As mentioned previously, community theatre is increasingly applied to diverse communities in non-traditional settings. For example, workshops for participants who have significant trust issues, such as youth in remand (i.e., corrections or juvenile detention) or domestic violence survivors, the opportunity to work collaboratively to achieve a common goal may facilitate change and help participants build trust. Theatre companies have also emerged for aspiring and emerging artists with disabilities who are offered professional training to enable them to earn income from their work. Participants gain a sense of self-worth and know that they are meaningfully contributing to the arts and broader community. For example in South Australia, *Tutti Arts,* is an "inclusive arts organisation...

which is dedicated to bringing people together through the arts without letting disability or disadvantage get in the way" (Tutti Arts, n.d.).

Like *Tutti Arts*, the highly acclaimed, award-winning *No Strings Attached: Theatre of Disability* (also based in South Australia) creates "original theatre through the unique perspectives of our disabled artists and performers" (No Strings Attached, 2014). The company tours nationally in Australia and conducts workshops that cater to the individual needs of participants. It produces world-class theatre, which both raises awareness for and about people with disability and supports members to "develop career paths in the performing arts" (No Strings Attached, 2014). The application of theatre to such a variety of situations requires that the practitioner be sensitive to the unique culture of each community group of participants.

Professional artists invited to facilitate community arts projects must therefore be prepared to adapt to each new culture. Established community groups will have their own norms, values, and beliefs. The artist will need to integrate into the community rather than adopt that community's culture. For example, facilitating an arts project with youth in remand or working within indigenous communities, the practitioner will consider their cultural background. Adopting mannerisms, speech, and habits would caricaturize their culture and disrespect or alienate participants. It is useful practice for both the practitioner and the community group to collaboratively develop an arts-related philosophy or value system specific to the project. This will assist the advancement of the project and help create a safe emotional space for the development of individuals' interpersonal skills. The project should recognise:

- The beliefs and values of individual participants;
- The cultural diversity of the group;
- The cultural heritage of individuals;
- The importance of equity and equality of ideas and values and their transmission;
- The importance of communication of differing points of view and those differences should be accepted, thus allowing for cultural democracy;
- The importance of self-identification, self-representation, and self-determination of the group; and
- The process, which creates a safe environment for democratic exchange of cultural expressions (Sue Harris Puppets, 1997).

These principles are important to both the process as well as the product of the endeavour when the community-developed philosophy is displayed within the theatre workshop space, it assists in creating a sense of belonging and helps maintain group unity.

Furthermore, the role of the practitioner is to assist the passage and progress of the art under construction. When working within a community (as opposed to creating the piece as voice for a culturally disadvantaged community), the practitioner must take care not to fall into the role of manager. As a specialist, the practitioner will direct and teach new skills; however, participants will ultimately create the art. For example, clients of Anglican Community Services selected puppetry to enact personal stories. Each had been in extreme situations of abuse, and the art form allowed participants to remain "one-step removed" from the actual experience. The theme for the vignettes was: "My life before intervention and my life and after intervention." Initially participants were introduced to the art of puppetry, given performance skills using large puppets, and then "let loose" with a pile of props. Scenarios gave health workers valuable feedback— affirmation that they were making a difference in the lives of people who, before intervention, considered themselves to be in situations with no hope for the future. Results were moving and empowering for participants and viewers of the performance. Each performance piece was created without dialogue so that those with limited articulation would feel included and empowered. The importance of clearly defined goals, interactive arts projects require specific parameters for the stability of the project and the emotional and physical safety of participants. Community theatre serves a cause; however, it also serves participants' development of interpersonal skills and growth.

Theatre, whether for community-cultural development, therapy, social action, education, or documentary has the ability to change the lives of participants, practitioner, and audience. The benefits of theatre include self and community empowerment, development of interpersonal skills, and growth and development including imagination, creativity, self-image, and self-confidence. Theatre provides a safe medium through which participants can give a voice to a range of personal and/or community issues. Issue-based theatre pieces developed by professional theatre makers for disadvantaged communities have the potential for broader community and health industry use. For example in the case study, *Perish the Thought* (2012), an edited video recording of the production is intended to become a useful adjunct for aged care, dementia care, carer support research with medical and health industry workers, and general public awareness and activism for social change.

One of the key challenges when considering the use of theatre in practice is funding. At the present time, a successful funding application often heavily relies on the ability to formulate an eloquent submission. Unless a community is self-funded, its art development may never eventuate. Government and corporate emphases influence funding decisions, which may impact on the development or style of the work. Questions arise such as: Will a community modify or alter its theatre piece in order to gain funding? If some aspect of the performance is significantly altered, how will this affect community ownership and morale? Will it change the focus of the message? How will this impact the project if there is a change or swing in community focus? Moreover, successful funding is often reliant on proving other economic or welfare benefits (Caust, 2003), which may require the practitioner to develop an evaluation of these endeavours.

Drama Therapy

Community theatre has broadened considerably in its application to diverse contexts. More than often community theatre practice inherently provides therapeutic benefits for the participants. However, it is important to note the development of drama therapy as a specialization, which offers an avenue for the use of theatrical performance for individuals and groups. Drama therapy seeks to achieve therapeutic outcomes through the use of drama (North American Drama

Therapy Association [NADTA], 2014). It can be used for the expressed purpose of storytelling, exploration of feelings, problem solving, catharsis, and interpersonal skill development (NADTA, 2014). The research regarding this approach continues to grow, and a number of studies show some promising results. For example, in a study of adult, male offenders in prison, drama therapy was combined with cognitive-behavioural techniques to determine if anger decreased from pre-test to post-test (Blacker, Watson, & Beech, 2008). Results indicated that significant reductions occurred and suggest that drama techniques may be a beneficial adjunct to traditional anger management programs (Blacker et al., 2008). A pilot study conducted with adults suffering from dementia was conducted with the use of drama and movement therapy. Qualitative results suggest that participants benefited from the program in terms of social interaction, both inside and outside the group; participants also indicated that they enjoyed their participation (Wilkinson, Srikumar, Shaw, & Orrell, 1998). In another pilot study, a school drama therapy intervention was employed as a preventive effort for emotional and behavioural issues and as a way to improve school performance for immigrant and refugee adolescents (Benoit et al., 2007). Following the 9-week intervention, participants in the drama therapy group (compared to those in the control group) showed lower levels of impairment and their math scores had significantly increased. These results suggest that drama therapy may be one way to intervene with adolescents who have complex emotional and social backgrounds (Benoit et al., 2007). Additional research is needed regarding the benefits and applications of drama therapy techniques in practice. For those who wish to use it in their practice, additional training in drama therapy is likely required in most countries, particularly for purposes of registration or accreditation. Educational programs, workshops, and trainings should be explored within the context of one's country of practice.

Ethical Considerations

Whose story are we telling and why? When interviews and life stories are told, ownership of the material is an important issue to consider. Clearly defined guidelines for copyright and intellectual property need to be in place before a project begins. There are Institutes of Arts Law and Arts Law Societies in United Kingdom, United States and Australia, which provide information sheets and advice. Relatedly, the issue of recompense, and sharing the proceeds is another topic for reflection. A community group's members will have differing ideologies and perceptions of events; therefore negotiation and communication are crucial to ensure equity amongst members.

Ethics in verbatim or documentary theatre is sometimes regarded as "too abstract and conceptual" (Gibson, 2011, p. 1); however, any interactive theatre project requires ethical considerations. The practitioner should consider the interrelationship of stories. In other words, all stories include and impact multiple individuals. We need to ask ourselves: What then is our responsibility to the other players in our life's story—or the story of the group? Heddon (2008) speaks to the topic of "the other"—our existence in relationship with others and the responsibilities it brings toward those "others" in the making of auto/biographical theatre (p.125). For example, if the theatre piece falls under the banner of social justice—who decides how much of the story will be told? Theatre makers should work closely with those who are the primary subject of the performance (e.g., victims of a crime, domestic violence survivors, children at risk, people with health issues) as well as relevant others (e.g., perpetrator of the crime/abuse, parents, carers) to carefully consider the motives for constructing the piece and any potential harm that might occur because of the way the story is told. Is the writing for personal notoriety or to give voice to the silent oppressed? Two-way communication between the participant and interviewer/playwright is imperative in the negotiation of subject matter and its disposal "because both lives and theatre-making practices are relational and transactional, and thus have an ethical dimension" (Gibson, 2011, p 6).

Case Example: Responsible Gambling Education

Facilitator: Susan Harris

This arts-based project occurred in Australia with students in their senior year of high school. Participants were Aboriginal students, and some were descendants of the "Stolen Generations."[54] Participants were drawn from two different high schools, both of which are situated in an area where problem gambling is common. This project was an adjunct to the *Responsible Gambling Education* program taught in Department for Education and Child Development (DECD) high schools in South Australia, and the project's life-span is on-going.

Participants' involvement in the initial project was about 30 hours in total, and the project is noteworthy as it raises some important issues both culturally and socially for facilitators of community theatre. Given their background and history, the group needed to "own" their workshop and performance space. Therefore, a supportive environment for participant learning and change was created so that students could take risks and explore their feelings, life-style, and attitudes. A graffiti wall, which was initially devised as a non-threatening means of gathering informal and honest feedback, became an intrinsic tool for staking ownership and brainstorming. Three events evolved:

1. Initially if a personal comment or feeling was inscribed, it would be tagged-over as protection to the writer. A rule of not tagging over graffiti was introduced after the second session. Each etching was sacred to its creator. Etchings had become the participants' "rock paintings" and as such needed to be respected and protected.
2. Students moved from tagging on the graffiti wall to using the markers to tag on the inside of windows. They reversed their art work in order for

---

[4] Stolen Generations: From the late 1800s to the 1970s many Aboriginal and some Torres Strait Islander children were forcibly removed from their families by past Australian Federal, State, and Territory governments and carried out by acts of parliament. Children were not permitted to visit their families and were sent either to institutions or adopted by non-indigenous families. For more information, see: http://www.nsdc.org.au/stolen-generations/history-of-the-stolen-generations/the-history-of-the-stolen-generations.

"outsiders" to be able to read the tags and know to whom the space belonged. They were consolidating their community.

3. It was a natural transition to use the "wall" during the brainstorming session for performance pieces. Students felt at ease with the space and added drawings to illustrate points where literacy skills were minimal.

Since participants came from different school environments, it was vital for the success of the project that a sense of familial belonging was created. As well as theatre sports and trust-related games, a story circle was formed where we met at the beginning and end of each session to plan, tell stories, and debrief as well as to brainstorm ideas and workshop philosophies.

Consideration for the personal history and self-esteem of participants was crucial for their well-being. For example, strict guidelines for participants, and the entire school community were firmly held. All visits by school staff members were limited, scheduled, and sanctioned by the entire group—the school principal included. However, it became evident to the facilitator from the outset that these students would not turn up on performance day if they felt pressured or coerced to perform. Although many of the students participating in the project had a history of non-attendance to regular lessons, they all attended every session and remained in our space for the entire school day. Instead of a live performance, we produced a DVD of participants' performances that could be used by the DECD. The students performed using glove puppets in order to retain anonymity and were proud to have their performances filmed and used for on-going efforts to assist other students.

Tips for Practitioners

1. **Planning, planning, and planning**. There can never be enough planning when undertaking a community theatre project and contingency plans should always be in place. For example, what happens if the funding is cut? Or what if participants decide not to participate?

2. **Begin with the goal and work backwards.** How many stages or steps will it take to achieve the goal? Be realistic in goal-setting and try to avoid over-extending yourself and your resources, including consideration if the goal is achievable in the time frame that you have available.

3. **Create equity between members.** By working collaboratively with participants, community members will know that their input is valued and important to the outcome.

4. **Allow for regular planning meetings and opportunities to debrief about the process.** These conversations should always hold the outcomes and philosophic base of the group in mind, but also create a space that allows for open exploration.

5. **When the project is over, allow for a grieving process**. Participants may feel a sense of loss when the project is over, and they will need a chance to express their grief.

6. **Stakeholders should know their responsibilities and be aware of funding criteria.** This will help ensure that the objectives of the project

are consistent with funding requirements, documentation of benchmarks are maintained to support those claims.

7. **All stakeholders should be familiar with the aims, outcomes, and community philosophy**. Participants should be aware of how the project will creatively demonstrate the community's vision of itself and feel comfortable with what will be shown to the audience.

8. **Plan for a celebration**. All projects come to an end, and it is important for participants to celebrate their achievements and growth as well as say farewell to the project.

9. **Think about the future**. What is next for the project or this community?

10. **Comprehensive documentation.** For archival purposes and future planning, documentation is important. Feedback on the project (verbal and/or written) from participants and audiences is useful in demonstrating the successful outcome(s) of the project.

Recommended Readings and Resources

Boal, A. (1992). *Games for actors and non-actors*. London: Routledge.

Emunah, R. (1994). *Acting for real: Drama therapy, process, technique, and performance*. New York: Brunner-Routledge.

Fo, D. (1991). *The tricks of the trade*. (Trans. J. Farrell). London: Methuen Drama.

Hazou, R. (2009). Refugee advocacy and the theatre of inclusion. *About Performance, 9*, 67-85.

Hawkins, G. (1993). *From Nimbin to Mardi Gras: Constructing community arts*. St. Leonards, New South Wales, Australia: Allen & Unwin.

Leonard, H., & Kilkelly, A. (2006). *Performing communities: Grassroots ensemble theaters deeply rooted in eight U.S. communities*. Oakland, CA: New Village Press.

Nicholson, H. (2005). *Applied drama: The gift of theatre*. New York: Plagrave MacMillan.

Pollock, D. (Ed.). (2005). *Remembering: Oral history performance*. Gordonsville, VA: Palgrave MacMillan.

Schweitzer, P. (2006). *Reminiscence theatre making theatre from memories*. London: Jessica Kingsley.

References

Australian Bureau of Statistics. (2012). Disability, ageing, and carers, Australia: Summary of the findings. Retrieved from: www.abs.gov.au/ausstats/abs@.nsf/Lookup/4430.0Chapter1102012.

Benoit, M., Gauthier, M. F., Lacroix, L., Alain, N., Rojas, M. V., Moran, A., & Bourassa, D. (2007). Classroom drama therapy for immigrant and refugee adolescents: A pilot study. *Clinical Child Psychology and Psychiatry, 12*(3), 451-465.

Blacker, J., Watson, A., & Beech, A. R. (2008). A combined drama-based and CBT approach to working with self-reported anger aggression. *Criminal Behaviour and Mental Health, 18*, 129-137.

Bottoms, S. (2006). Putting the document into documentary. *TDR: The Drama Review, 50*(3), 56-68.

Brook, P. (1968). *The Empty Space*. London: Penguin Books.

Capelin, S. (Ed.). (1995). *Challenging the centre: Two decades of political theatre*. Brisbane: Playlab Press.

Caust, J. (2003). Putting the "art" back into arts policy making: How arts policy has been "captured" by the economists and the marketers. *The International Journal of Cultural Policy, 9*(1), 51-63.

Enright, N. (1996). *Blackrock*. Sydney: Currency Press.

Gibson, J. (2011). *Saying it right: Creating ethical verbatim theatre*. Retrieved from:
http//arts.mq.edu.au/documents/har_journal_neo/neoJanet2011_2_pdf.

Hage, G. (2003). *Against paranoid nationalism: Searching for hope in a shrinking society*. Australia: Pluto Press.

Heddon, D. (2008). *Autobiography and performance*. Basingstoke: Palgrave Macmillan.

Kershaw, B. (1992). *The politics of performance: Radical theatre as cultural intervention*. London: Routledge.

McCallum, J. (2006). A certain maritime incident: Introduction. *Australasian Drama Studies, 48*, 136-142.

Martin, C. (2006). Bodies of evidence. *TDR: The Drama Review, 50*(3), 8-15.

National Sorry Day Committee. (n.d.). *Stolen generations*. Retrieved from: http://www.nsdc.org.au/stolen-generations/history-of-the-stolen-generations/the-history-of-the-stolen-generations.

No Strings Attached: Theatre of Disability. (2014). *About us*. Retrieved from: http://www.nostringsattached.org.au/about-us.html.

North American Drama Therapy Association [NADTA]. (2014). *What is drama therapy?* Retrieved from: www.nadta.org/what-is-drama-therapy.html.

Prendergast, M., & Saxton, J. (Eds.). (2009). *Applied theatre international case studies and challenges for practice*. Bristol: Intellect.

Prentki, T., & Preston, S., (Eds.). (2009). *The applied theatre reader*. Oxon, UK: Routledge.

Reinelt, J. (2006). Toward a poetics of theatre and public events. *TDR: The Drama Review, 50*(3), 69-83.

South Australian Department for Education and Child Development. (2010). Retrieved from: http:www.decd.sa.gov/policy/pages/OSPP/policy.

Sue Harris Puppets. (1997). *Philosophic base for Project Work with children*. Retrieved from: www.sueharris.com.au.

Svich, C. (2003). Moises Kaufman: Reconstructing history through theatre: An Interview. *Contemporary Theatre Review, 13*(3), 67-72.

Tutti Arts. (n.d.). *Tutti Arts*. Retrieved from: http://tutti.org.au/.

Wilkinson, N., Srikumar, S., Shaw, K., & Orrell, M. (1998). Drama and movement therapy in dementia: A pilot study. *The Arts in Psychotherapy, 25*(3), 195-201.

Willet, J. (Ed. & Trans.). (1982). *Brecht on theatre*. London: Eyre Methuen.

Chapter 13: Reflections of Me: How Visual Storytelling is Changing How We Interact with the World

Wilson Main & Carolyn Bilsborow

People are happier, more engaged with the world, and more likely to develop or learn, when they are doing and making things for themselves, rather than having things done and made for them (Gauntlett, 2011, p. 226).

Introduction

In years to come, we may look back on the twentieth century as an anomaly in human history, not because of the wars, which engulfed the entire world, nor because of our first steps on the moon, but because of the way large corporations of professional media-makers hijacked our channels of communication and storytelling. Prior to the emergence of the newspaper, radio, cinema, and television industries, the stories we told each other were ours; they were local and personal, and they were expressions of our own personal creativity. Then, Hollywood, the BBC, Disney, and Fox, to name but a few, re-packaged our stories into universally appealing themes, polished them with magic, and sold them back to us through our newspapers, radios, television, and cinema screens.

Prior to our entrancement by mass media, we had a history of personal creative expression, which sadly many of us forgot as we sat down to watch *Lost in Space* or *Neighbours* each night. But now, in the dawn of the digital and social media environment, we not only have the opportunity to tell our own stories once again, but also for the first time in human history we have the ability to access tools for visual storytelling. This technology has become so ubiquitous that it is profoundly changing the way that we interact with the world. With its availability, affordability, and ease of use, digital media has provided communities and individuals with the capacity to be creators and broadcasters of their own stories once again, now told powerfully through the medium of the moving image.

Social media commentator Clay Shirky identifies that while people like to consume media they also have a desire to produce and share it. Shirky (2010) argues that traditional 20th Century mass media was run as a single event—consumption. Traditional mass media could talk to us, but we could not talk to it. As the 20th Century wore on, many of us spent the hours that would have once been spent being creative, used that time to watch or read mass media. Now, in the emergent digital and social media environment, we find ourselves able to not only consume media, but also create and share our personal messages to the world.

The tools of production for film and TV communication have rested for almost a century in the hands of the media elite. Production equipment was heavy, cumbersome, expensive, and beyond the reach of most people. The barriers to entry were profound, and the power to disseminate our cultural stories lay in the hands of those who could afford the equipment, the wages, and had control the distribution of product. Many, although not all, of those barriers, particularly the technological and distribution barriers, have vanished in the late 2000s.

Buckingham, Harvey, and Sefton-Green (1999) lauded the value of the new digital production tools to students, but lamented the limited means of distribution for such products. Six years later, this problem had been solved with the arrival of the new video sharing sites of which YouTube has become the most prominent. YouTube was more than happenstance; it was inevitable. Winston (2002) argued that new innovations are not driven by new technology and only leave the theoretical or prototype stage when they meet a "supervening social necessity." According to Winston (2002), new, technologically based products are a result of society's needs rather than the technology itself being the generator of new desires and behaviours. YouTube broke the dams of "walled-in" creativity that had been previously constrained by the need of broadcasters and studios, bound by enormous technology and production expenses, forced to reject non-mass market, niche products because they were not commercially viable. Now everyone can not only produce, but also broadcast. The floodgates have opened, and we witnessed some new phenomena including videologs (vlogs), fan produced media, including feature length films, citizen journalism, community productions, consumer protest videos, and much more.

We are not underestimating the value of technical or analytical skills, but rather we are celebrating that for the first time in history the ability to tell "filmic" stories has been delivered to the community at large. For the first time, the technology is approaching invisibility and the barriers to its use are low. In this chapter, the emphasis is on the skills of producing content; that is, telling a story, rather than the mastery of technology.

The Creative Journey of Visual Storytelling

The motivation to make a visual story is often driven by the desire to have a finished story to show others, but the process of actually creating the story can also be a rich and rewarding journey. Training people to tell visual stories requires them to choose a subject, usually based on a fact that they are passionate about, and embark on a journey of discovery in search of the pieces of the puzzle.

> The process of making is enjoyed for its own sake, of course: there is pleasure in seeing a project from start to finish, and the process provides space for thought and reflection, and helps to cultivate a sense of the self as an active, creative agent. But there is also a desire to connect and communicate with others and—especially online—to be an active participant in dialogues and communities (Gauntlett, 2011, p. 222).

Methodologically, creating visual stories can be likened to practice-based research or learning where the experience of the journey is as valuable as the outcomes. This section will discuss the practice-based learning methodology that underlies visual storytelling and the benefits of understanding the process of creating self-made media.

Visual storytelling has close ties to documentary or factual production, and the most fundamental definition of documentary reveals that the genre attempts to represent natural (factual or "real") elements of the world for the purpose of allowing the world to see itself (Grierson, 1946). Contemporary documentary producers such as Michael Moore place themselves at the centre of their inquiry into the "natural" world and their resulting "reports" (the documentary or visual story) offer the multiple realities that the filmmaker encountered during the inquiry. The art of visual storytelling is thus collaborative, creative, complex, and emergent. It allows the storyteller to create their own perspective of a world and then reflect on their position in that world.

Tacit Knowledge

> Since creative arts research is often motivated by emotional, personal, and subjective concerns, it operates not only on the basis of explicit and exact knowledge, but also on that of tacit knowledge (Barrett & Bolt, 2007, p. 4).

In visual storytelling, personal interest and experience motivate the production process and are the primary sources of innovation and new knowledge. The knowledge underlying this personal interest and experience can be thus described as tacit knowledge: the additional, often unconscious thought that accompanies explicit knowledge when put into action.

Polanyi (1966) defines tacit knowledge as the relationship between the theoretical aspect of knowledge or "knowing what" and the practical aspect of knowledge or "knowing how." Polanyi (1966) argues that things cannot just be observed and be thoroughly known and understood, they must be experienced. He explains, "it is not by looking at things, but by dwelling in them, that we can understand their joint meaning" (p. 18). Given that a practice-based process, such as visual storytelling, is focussed upon insights arising from making something, it is important to acknowledge these two aspects of knowing (*knowing what* and *knowing how*) and the relationship that exists between them. The activity of practicing anything allows the researcher to bring together and dwell in the two identified aspects of knowledge. Practice leads to an *interiorisation* of the knowledge and this process creates a tacit knowing. Creating visual stories allows the storyteller a deep immersion into both the creative process and a deeper understanding of the subject being explored.

The Storyteller is Central to the Process

Dewey (1958) clearly articulates the important role of the self:

> Experience is a matter of the interaction of organism with its environment...the organism brings with it through its own structure, native and acquired, forces that play a part in the interaction. The self acts...and its undergoings are not impressions stamped upon an inert wax but depend upon the way the organism reacts and responds. There is no experience in which human contribution is not a factor in determining what actually happens (p. 246).

As soon as "I" the storyteller step into the visual story production, every minute detail of the project alters in relationship to me. The social, cultural, political, and ideological make-up of the storyteller constructs the recursive formula that produces the visual story. Visual storytelling in the digital and social media environment allows us to return to the local and personal stories that we have told for centuries, only now, we can share them with the world.

The Role of the Audience

Over the last decade we have seen a shift from a passive viewing audience to an interactive user in terms of media consumption. The once-mass audience is now considered fragmented, individualised, and personalised. This section discusses the position held by the audience in either traditional broadcast or mass media era and in the contemporary digital era.

The Traditional Media Audience

In traditional or pre-digital media studies, there is a long, well-documented history of audience study approaches; all differ in the amount of power or activity that is afforded to the audience. Beginning in the 1930s with Effects Theory, the *hypodermic model* was developed out of the Frankfurt School of Social Research. This perspective presumed that the message sent by the producer of the media would be passively and naïvely accepted by each member of that audience. Ideas could simply be injected into viewers as if by a hypodermic needle. Over the next sixty years various other perspectives on the mass audience emerged with each succession affording more power to the audience.

The Digital Media-User

While traditional media audiences largely had only the power to consume media as it was delivered to them, the digital media user now has the power to create and share it. The digital media user is no longer being written about as a passive watcher, but rather, as an active creator, a sharer, a member of communities, and an expresser of life (Bruns, 2009; Jenkins, 2006; Gauntlett, 2011; Shirky, 2010). Since the early 1990s, Henry Jenkins (1992a; 1992b; 2003; 2006; 2009) has been examining both traditional and digital media users and the ways in which they participate with media, particularly in terms of fan culture; that is, fans creating media related to their interest in a specific professional production. Jenkins and others (Gauntlett, 2011; Shirky, 2010) acknowledge that people were creating their own media long before the emergence of Web 2.0 technologies:

> YouTube does not so much change the conditions of production as it alters the contexts of circulation and reception. Such works now reach a larger public via its channels of distribution; there are systems of criticism which focus attention on interesting and emerging works; there are people willing to seek out and engage with non-commercial content, and consumers are conversing with each other by producing videos (Burgess & Green, 2009, p. 113).

It is useful to examine how and why people enjoy being creative as a means for understanding the motivations for producing digital media. Csikszentmihalyi (1996) and Gardner (1993) have explored the experience of creativity and determined that those throughout history who have been considered as "creative" have successfully brought together three elements: the individual (their skills and talent); the domain of knowledge that the individual works in; and the field or the gatekeepers that work in the domain where the individual works (Csikszentmihalyi, 1996; Gardner, 1993). Gauntlett (2007) refers to this system of creativity as a "creative triangle." Without a connection between all three, an individual's creativity may go unnoticed. In a more recent work, Gauntlett (2011) furthers this definition of creativity for the digital realm. Everyday creativity refers to a process, which brings together at least one active human mind, and the material or digital world, in the activity of making something, which is novel in that context, and is a process, which evokes a feeling of joy (Gauntlett, 2011, p. 221).

More recently, attention has begun to turn to the act of digital media users being creative (Bruns, 2009; Gauntlett, 2011; Shirky, 2010). Gauntlett (2011) identifies a recent shift towards a "making and doing" culture, which incorporates "creativity, social connections, and personal growth" (p. 8). Gauntlett (2011) summarises five key principles related to digital media users' creativity: 1) a new understanding of creativity as process, emotion, and presence; 2) the drive to make and share; 3) happiness through creativity and community; 4) a middle layer of creativity as social glue; and 5) making your mark and making the world on your own. Shirky (2010), writing in the context of the development of *Wikipedia,* concentrates on identifying how the drive to create and share digital media has emerged. He suggests that there is a cognitive surplus, which he describes as the free time of the world's educated citizens that, in the past, has been invested in watching television but is now being focused on creating and sharing digital media.

The Importance of Storytelling

Many writers have argued that stories are fundamental to the human experience and critical to our psychological well-being (Campbell, 1949; Bettleheim, 1976; Booker, 2004). Through the stories told by our ancestors, parents, and peers, we come to understand, as the ancient Greeks wrote, how we should live our lives. The Lumiere Brothers in 1895 gave storytelling a new dimension when they managed to popularise the technique of information transfer through the moving image. The new medium of film was more than simply information or entertainment novelty. The eventual addition of actors, sound, music, colour, animation, and sophistication, although highly succinct, storytelling structures created powerful emotional experiences that allowed a more intense degree of vicarious identification with the protagonists and antagonists that populated these tales. It could move audiences to laughter or tears, and it also had the power to persuade and affect human behaviours. The Lumiere Brothers first works were called "actualities." A camera fixed to a tripod pointed at an actual event–a train rushing by, workers leaving a factory or the Melbourne Cup horse race in Australia. Today, modern "actualities" or documentaries can be more than the transmission of facts. They can offer engaging or moving stories of humans engaged in extraordinary experiences and provide an emotional communication tool for a community organization. Whether those emotions are empathy, sadness, humour, or joy, they have the power to change awareness. But more importantly, they have the power to change attitudes and beliefs.

Documentary is personal truth

Documentary has a relationship with the factual, but it should not be seen as "truth." Rather it is a highly subjective "truth" as seen through the eyes of a director who chooses which subjects to interview, which camera angles to use, and selectively edits what has been filmed. S/he chooses the music, graphics, vision, and constructs the story that s/he wants to tell. A tacit agreement exists with the audience that the film is providing an account of reality that is based in facts and evident, and the audience will know if that agreement is dishonored (Stevens, 2009). While this idea of truth may be subjective, many documentary makers do argue that they are striving to show an authentic truth.

Empathy

In an age where connection and empathy is decreasing (Konrath, O'Brien, Hsing, 2011; Twenge, 2013), stories may be a solution to the problem of fostering empathic growth and positive social behaviours in places where they seem to be lacking. This could include offenders or those who live in places where parties are in conflict or even where fear or unjustified disdain for "the other" is manifest. In teaching participants to research, understand, and then tell the stories of others, we are also teaching empathy.

Johnson (2012) argues that narrative fiction fosters empathic growth and an understanding of the social world. Stories allow us to compress, simplify, and abstract the complexities of community living and human interaction. Stories presented on the screen take us into the worlds of others and allow us to live for a time in a simulated world where we can vicariously experience the physical and internal world of actors whose on screen lives become metaphors for our own. To create factual stories also requires empathic observation as a key skill set of the filmmaker.

A Means to Teach, Persuade, or Disseminate Information

McLuhan (1968) espouses that the tribal campfire as a scene of group connections and storytelling has now been replaced by the blue glow of the television set. As ever, human beings crave the stories of our tribal members; it is only the delivery mechanism that changes. These tales are more than mere entertainment. Stories provide repositories of knowledge for mankind that increases the ability for our species to survive (Dutton, 2005).

Human beings make sense of their environment through stories as metaphors, pattern recognition and completion, learning to plan, and organising their behaviours. Art allows us to problem solve and ponder different ways to address our problems or issues (Dutton, 2005). Through the process of learning to produce visual stories, participants are gaining both reasoning and communication skills. Every story contains a message whether one intends it or not. Once we place a frame around a visual we are saying "look at this, it is important." The filmmaker controls this and thus must learn the skills of visual communication, but also the skills of argument, persuasion, and reasoning.

Producing Digital Stories as Therapy

Theorists of filmmaking have often explored the relationship between film and psychology (Metz, 1974, 1982; Mulvey, 1975). Johnson and Anderson (2008) sought to take this further and explore the use of filmmaking as therapy taken from the client's perspective. Combining a number of elements including narrative therapy, art, and talk, they additionally provided the means by which three patients would film and edit their own productions outside of their regular therapy sessions. The topics were left open, and the only condition was that it should be related to their reason for seeking therapy. After a three-week period the films would be transcribed, analysed, and discussed with the researchers. The therapy provided a number of positive advantages including feelings of mastery and changed perceptions of self and others in particular situations. The camera allowed them to view the objective nature of the camera's revelations against their own subjective perceptions.

In another example, O'Rourke (2001) describes the use of video therapy in treating trauma with child war survivors. She described how the victims see their traumatic memories as moving pictures over which they have no control. She describes the reaction of a girl named Anya by using video. With its ability to stop and start, the child gradually began to feel a sense of mastery over her own internal images. Children are often challenged by verbal expression of their feelings and thoughts, especially the nightmares and traumatic memories that are associated with psychological trauma. Film can provide an outlet for those difficult thoughts and feelings in a visual format, which can allow survivors to create an account of their experience, monitor their reactions to environmental stimuli, and over time, control their emotional responses. Moreover, when children are allowed to act as the both the subject and director of their own film, they can work toward moving past their traumatic past and see themselves in a new light—as moviemakers (O'Rourke, 2001). If the film is shared with an audience, survivors gain an opportunity to be heard.

In addition, film may also be used therapeutically for prevention and intervention efforts in myriad ways. For example, a 35-minute documentary-type film was created called *Lead with Love*, which was aimed at parents of lesbian, gay, or bisexual children and provided information and ways for them to support their children (view for free at: www.leadwithlovefilm.com/film.html). Data from a follow-up study indicates that parents' sense of self-efficacy improved as a result of viewing the film (Huebner, Rullo, Thoma, McGarrity, & Mackenzie, 2013). In another prevention-intervention type approach to film-making, four African American women who are HIV+ created a documentary on the "dark side" of HIV. The film that they created is meant to be shown to adolescent females with the goal of increasing education and reducing sexual risk-taking behaviors; however, in a study of the film-makers response to the making of the film, the results reveal that the women gained self-acceptance, felt liberated by self-disclosing their HIV+ status, garnered support from the other women involved in the project, and felt that film would help others avoid what they had experienced (Norris & DeMarco, 2005). This dual purpose of film for intervention and prevention offers another way to conceive of using film for therapeutic purposes.

Benefits and Potential Challenges

We are living in a new media landscape, one that can include everyone as both producers of visual stories and also distributors of those stories. Profound new uses of the media are being explored as new innovations are presented to us daily and as we are remembering our role as storytellers. Creative works can have a powerful effect on the storytellers as they investigate and tell the stories that are important to them as well as the audiences that view them. Filmmaking can allow participants to rediscover their creativity and promote community interaction to rebuild that which is being lost.

Film offers a unique opportunity for self-expression, one that combines the power of storytelling with new media. Not only is the technology increasingly available to massive amounts of people, but also it is relatively cheap, making it even more accessible. Thus, filmmaking can offer a wide range of applications for practice, particularly for adolescents and young adults who are wired. However, the assumption that young people, who find it easy to use the digital technology and have grown up with vast quantities of media at their fingertips, will know how to take the new, readily accessible tools of production and turn them into powerful dramas or documentaries is one that should be held lightly. Technology is only a mechanism. The real motivation is not to merely undertake a technical operation to perfectly capture images and sound, but rather to satisfy a desire to say something about human nature, values, and interactions that when encapsulated in powerful stories provides us with an interpretation of the world that the filmmaker wishes the viewer to share.

Filmmaking allows for mass communication of a particular perspective, issue, or story, which has the power to reach a lot of people quickly. Images are powerful, and films offer a new and exciting opportunity to work with communities large and small. For example, a group of filmmakers may want to show how their community exhibits certain strengths and issues. Such a film could then be used to create further dialogue about change within the community—both amongst its members as well as those who are positions of power.

One of the challenges of filmmaking is that participants may not be representing "reality" in quite the way that they imagined. In fact, they are likely presenting a perspective on truth, which is not so much a challenge per se, but something that should be considered during the process. Another key challenge relates to the age and experience that participants have with the filmmaking process. Young filmmakers are relatively new to the world of adulthood and their existing knowledge and frameworks for how they see the world and others may be undeveloped. They may not possess the confidence to approach potential interviewees. Similarly, they may make the assumption that all adults are "adult" (i.e., mature, confident, all knowing). They do not understand that these "adults" are often more like them, and thus have some trepidation about asking them difficult questions. Practice and experience with interviewing will help young (or new) filmmakers ask better questions, be present in the moment, and gain confidence through the process.

Ethical Considerations

As filmmakers, we construct highly edited images and stories involving individuals. Many issues of representation are obvious; sexism, racism, and ageism amongst others are clearly to be avoided. As Rabiger (2009) states "[obvious ethical] clarity is rare; usually it's not black-and-white issues we deal with but shades of grey" (p. 344).

Stephen Carthew, a colleague, was involved with an alternative spiritual group in the 1970s in Western Australia. The documentary program *Compass* produced a history of the group titled *The Brotherhood,* and Carthew participated generously, eagerly looking forward to the program's broadcast. To his surprise, when it played nationally on the ABC (Australian Broadcasting Commission), he was portrayed as a manipulative cult leader who had damaged people's lives. Carthew argues that not revealing the intent of the story direction was deceptive and unethical on the part of the producers, and the ramifications for Carthew and others who appeared in the documentary are still being felt four years on. Similarly, Rabiger (2009) cites the case of a factory worker who spoke candidly about the sexual morals of her co-worker while on film. When it was broadcast, her co-workers were furious and beat her up. Therefore, upfront discussions regarding the potential ramifications of the film should be explored with participants.

Moreover, interviewers, in an attempt to relate to the human being sitting in front of them, will nod and smile, encouraging them to talk further. Respected documentarian Albert Maysles (2009) emphasises the importance of being an observer. Such behaviour can be read by the interviewee as indicating agreement and as empathy with their position. Extremes are to be avoided–being too empathic or not empathic at all. Maysles (2009) argues that the interviewer should not judge, but rather reveal to the audience and allow them to decide. However, this is not a universally adopted principle, and some interviewers, such as Michael Moore, often take an opinionated, subjective stance.

Case Application: Teaching Visual Storytelling

These case studies are drawn from a filmmaking course that is taught as a first year course in the undergraduate degree Bachelor of Media Arts at the University of South Australia. While this is a university-based course held over a 13-week period, the practical application is congruent with visual storytelling workshops conducted in any environment, and the structure can be condensed to fit a workshop of any duration.

Participants were required to meet with each other and their instructor on a weekly basis. During these meetings, teams had the opportunity to organise the project and discuss the story development with their tutor/instructor. Providing participants with adequate time and space to discuss their progress with either peers or the facilitator is essential.

During these sessions, it often became apparent that while students had successfully gathered the facts of the story, they had not explored the implications or over-arching themes behind the stories. We encouraged the students to explore these deeper meanings underpinning the stories to create a more engaging experience for the audience. An essential element to this process is self-reflection, and we ask the students to reflect, not only on their own process, but also on their peers. Being able to see and evaluate where they have been on a creative journey can be both life enhancing and therapeutic. As discussed earlier in the chapter, the process of making stories is as important as showing the finished product to others.

Case Study 1

Wendy (her Anglicised nom-de plume) is a 23-year-old girl from North Vietnam who is studying in Australia. She found that Australians were very different to what she had learned growing up in Vietnam. She had thought of Australians and Americans as being virtually interchangeable. They had been the invaders of her country during the Vietnam War. She produced a documentary interviewing her father who was a soldier for the North and Australian veterans who had fought during that war. From the beginning, we advised her that the film would be more powerful if she could interview both sides. The result is a highly moving documentary in which both sides talk honestly and with considerable insight into their personal experiences. It is a powerful anti-war statement that resolves many of Wendy's questions about the war. It will also have resonance for both Australian and North Vietnam veterans.

Excerpt from Wendy's Self-Evaluation

"In the first interview, we met with Michael H. and his girlfriend in a cafe for a pre-interview. It did not go well, and I questioned my ability. On the actual day of the shoot, he answered totally differently. He was more emotional and willing to share valuable information. I realised that he did not want to admit what he truly thought in front of his girlfriend. Next time, if I pre-interview someone who has a sensitive story, I will definitely meet them alone. It is an easier way to convince people to share their stories."

Case Study 2

One of our student teams asked a technically skilled young man who had extensive knowledge in camera and lighting techniques to work with them. He immediately had an idea that sounded exciting to the team. His plan was that they film a young Hollywood actor that he knew through a family connection. The actor was returning to his hometown and staying nearby with his family between films. The tutor questioned the wisdom of this and asked for their proposed narrative. Was there a story here or was it merely a profile of someone famous? The young man argued vociferously and took the team on a long and ultimately fruitless journey. What should have been an enriching journey typical to the visual storytelling process became a stressful and emotionally unsatisfying experience. They constructed a star profile. It looked great, but had nothing to say. It was pretty, but dreary.

There are three lessons here. Firstly, the value of collaboration with people who share the same values and who communicate positively cannot be underestimated. Secondly, without a story or point of view, a film can be a pointless exercise. Thirdly, technical skills are valuable to have, no question, but they are always trumped by the ability to tell a great story.

Tips for Practitioners

1. **Place a large emphasis on research.** This can be the longest part of the documentary process. Spend time with the participants discussing the possible stories that have emerged from what they found. Challenge their subjective assumptions and encourage them to think objectively and critically abut the subject matter.
2. **Ask participants to develop a point of view or a hypothesis.** What footage/interviews will they need to obtain to achieve their aim? Why do they feel compelled to present this viewpoint? What is the larger meaning?
3. **Emphasise that documentaries require more than just facts.** Correcting facts or misconceptions is not an effective tool of persuasion, but rather "individuals who receive unwelcome information may not simply resist challenges to their views. Instead, they may come to support their original opinion even more strongly—what they call a 'backfire effect'" (Nyan & Rieflerb, 2010, p. 307). Stories that show catharsis and emotion are far more powerful than making factual arguments. Make your audience *feel* something.
4. **Remember: this is *visual* storytelling.** Often, participants will focus on who to interview and which parts of the interview to use. This can result in a story that contains endless talking, and it is exhausting for the

viewer to watch. It is also inefficient in terms of communicating the story. The old adage, "a picture paints a thousand words," is true. Using a montage of music and pictures interlaced with talking-heads is a far more dynamic approach to visual storytelling. It also allows the viewer space to reflect on what is being said if there are breaks in the verbal storytelling.

5. **Music conveys emotion and sets the pace.** Choosing the right music to use is imperative to the desired message being conveyed by the visual story. A dynamic banjo-based instrumental track will convey a completely different message from a gentle, flowing orchestral track, and so the storyteller should decide what emotion they are attempting to communicate. Is this an uplifting, dramatic, horrific, or pensive story? Choosing the wrong piece of music can be likened to having a conversation with your best-friend by shouting aggressively at them … it can have disastrous effects.

6. **Planning on paper is important!** For a professional production, the initial pre-production planning stage is essential to communicating an engaging story. Pre-production paperwork is often used to sell an idea or story to help raise funds for a production. However, in a community-based production you will need to decide whether you have the time to include this stage because it can be a lengthy process.

7. **Choose an interesting environment.** Avoid filming people against bland white walls. Pick an environment that says something about your theme. If it is a cluttered environment, try to make sure that nothing appears to be growing out of the interviewee's head and that the background is not distracting.

8. **Avoid shooting against bright windows.** This will make your subject appear in silhouette. The key principle is that we want to see the subject's face and natural skin tones. You can bounce light off a ceiling, wall, or white surface of any kind onto your subject to create a soft lighting effect. After you have achieved your primary goal, you can check if there is anything else in this environment that it is important to see, and try to correct it if it is underlit. There are many lighting tutorials available on YouTube. Lighting does not have to be expensive or complicated.

9. **Good sound is crucial.** Turn off air-conditioners and ask neighbours to turn off their lawnmowers while you get the shot. Avoid environments with too much room reverberation. Get your microphone in as close as possible to the source of sound. The camera microphone is rarely good enough, especially if the camera is some distance away, so think about using an external microphone.

10. **Think about how you frame your subject.** Do not be afraid of getting the camera in close, especially if it is an emotional topic. The old hunting adage works for video as well – "don't shoot until you see the whites of their eyes." Many beginners shoot very wide, and this loses a great deal of impact.

Tips for Interviewing

Interviewing is a common element in producing visual stories. It requires active listening skills and planned, directed questioning. In the documentary series *Capturing Reality* (2009), Maysles claims that human beings have a need to disclose. Errol Morris (2009), also a pioneering documentary filmmaker, instructs us to stop talking and listen. Most participants will already be familiar with the idea of "open" and "closed" questions. The oft-stated theory that open questions invite expansive answers and that closed questions invite frustrating yes/no answers is not necessarily true in practice given that subjects have usually agreed to be involved.

Silence is also a great questioning tool. If the interviewee stays silent, then the interviewer can demonstrate they are listening with appropriate body language or nodding, which often encourages the subject to expand on what s/he is saying. A much greater challenge is getting beyond the facts to understand the issues behind the facts. A recent instance from a filmmaking course is illustrative. A middle-aged male interviewee declares to an amateur interviewer that he lost his position as a prominent newsreader when the television station decided they wanted to hire only attractive young, female presenters and that they no longer wanted old grey haired men like himself. Personal and emotional issues abound here but the interviewer, not listening, goes back to his list of questions and asks the next—and entirely unrelated—fact-based question.

The audience is not engaged in a quest for facts, but rather a quest for understanding through the elements of story and meaningful revelation. Facts are necessary and assist in placing the viewer inside the world of the subject, but they are not enough. They need to be placed "inside" the experience of the subject. The result is an interview that can feel more like a dinner party conversation than a story with the power to move, influence, or persuade us.

We use a three level approach to teach interviewing skills (see Figure 1). Note that these stages are not chronological, but rather they are types of questions, all of which are necessary to the interview. They can occur at any time, but are more likely to occur in the following order:

1. *The factual question.* What? How? When? Where?
2. *The implication question.* This is an exploration of deeper meaning and may include emotional consequences. Questions/responses would include: "Why?" "Tell me more." "That must have caused some problems for you." For example, the participant may be interviewing an over-zealous record collector who has run up debt and completely taken over the family home with his obsession. In this level you may ask: "How does your family feel about your entire house being filled with Vinyl LPs?" "How do your children feel about not being able to bring home friends?"
3. *Empathetic questions.* In level three, a sense of understanding and meaning in the story we are telling is necessary. Questions/responses may include:
   - How did that make you feel?
   - That must have been awful for you.
   - Was that tough to go through?
   - You really feel strongly about this, don't you?

- What will it mean to you if you don't get help/achieve this?
- Why do you think people collect things? Why are they so important to you? What does collecting mean to you?
- How do you feel about your children's reaction to my earlier question?
- Some people might suggest that this is a very selfish pursuit. How would you answer them?

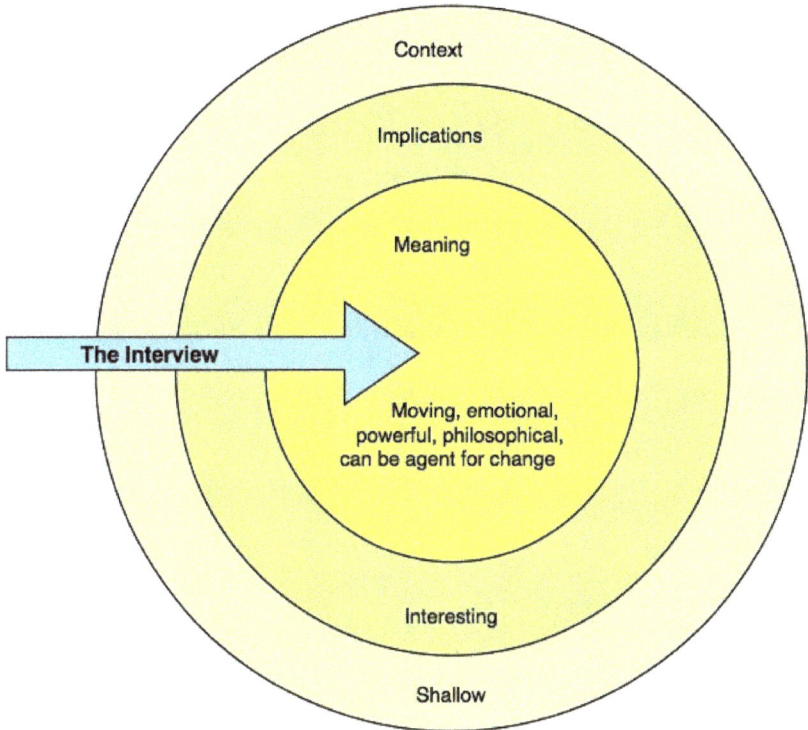

Context

Implications

Meaning

The Interview

Moving, emotional, powerful, philosophical, can be agent for change

Interesting

Shallow

© Wilson Main 2013

Figure 1

Recommended Readings and Resources

Beusekom, M. V., Ferrari, P., & Baichwal, J. (2009). *Capturing reality: The art of documentary*. New York: First Run Features.

Gauntlett, D. (2011). *Making is connecting*. United Kingdom: Polity Press.

Lambert, J. (2013). *Digital storytelling: Capturing lives, creating community* (4th ed.) New York: Routledge.

Rabiger, M. (2009). *Directing the documentary* (5th ed.). Boston, MA: Focal Press.

Shirky, C. (2010). *Cognitive surplus: Creativity and generosity in a connected age*. New York: Penguin.

References

Barrett, E., & Bolt, B. (2007). *Practice as research: Approaches to creative arts enquiry.* New York: Palgrave Macmillan.

Bettelheim, B. (1976). *The uses of enchantment: The meaning and importance of fairy tales.* New York: Random House.

Booker, C. (2004). *The seven basic plots: Why we tell stories.* London: Continuum.

Bruns, A. (2009). *Blogs, Wikipedia, second life, and beyond: From production to produsage.* New York: Peter Lang Publishing.

Buckingham, D., Harvey, I., & Sefton-Green, J. (1999). Convergence. *The International Journal of Research into New Media Technologies, 5,* 10-20.

Burgess, J., & Green J. (2009). *YouTube: Digital media and society series.* United Kingdom: Polity Press.

Campbell, J. (1949). *The hero with a thousand faces.* Princeton, NJ: Princeton University Press.

Csikszentmihalyi, M. (1996). *Creativity.* New York: Harper Perennial.

Dewey, J. (1958). *Art as experience* (9th ed.). New York: Capricorn Books.

Dutton, D. (2005). Authenticity and art. In J. Levinson (Ed.), *The Oxford handbook for aesthetics* (pp. 258-274). New York: Oxford University Press.

Gardener, H. (1993). *Creating minds: An anatomy of creativity seen through the lives of Freud, Einstein, Picasso, Stravinksy, Eliot, Graham and Gandhi.* New York: Basic Books.

Gauntlett, D. (2007). *Creative explorations: New approaches to identities and audiences.* London: Routledge.

Gauntlett, D. (2011). *Making is connecting.* United Kingdom: Polity Press.

Grierson, J. (1946). *Grierson on documentary.* F. Hardy (Ed.). New York: Praeger Publishers.

Huebner, D. M., Rullo, J. E., Thoma, B. C., McGarrity, L. A., & Mackenzie, J. (2013). Piloting *Lead with Love*: A film-based intervention to improve parents' response to their lesbian, gay, and bisexual children. *Journal of Primary Prevention, 34,* 359-369.

Jenkins, H. (2006). *Convergence culture: Where old and new media collide.* New York: New York University Press.

Johnson, J. L., & Alderson, K. G. (2008). Therapeutic filmmaking: An exploratory pilot study. *The Arts in Psychotherapy, 35,* 11-19.

Johnson, D. R. (2012). Transportation into a story increases empathy, prosocial behavior, and perceptual bias toward fearful expressions. *Personality and Individual Differences, 52,* 150.

Konrath, S. H., O'Brien, E. H., & Hsing, C. (2011). Changes in dispositional empathy in American college students over time: A meta-analysis. *Personality and social psychology review: An official Journal of the Society for Personality and Social Psychology, 15,* 180-198.

Maysles, A. (2009). Interview. In M. V. Beusekom, P. Ferrari, & J. Baichwal (Eds.), *Capturing reality: The art of documentary.* New York: First Run Features.

McLuhan, M. (1968). *War and peace in the global village.* New York: Bantam.

Metz, C. (1974). *Film language: A semiotics of the cinema*. New York: Oxford University Press.

Metz, C. (1982). *The imaginary signifier: Psychoanalysis and the cinema* (translated by C. Britton, A. Williams, B. Brewster, & A. Guzzetti). Bloomington, IN: Indiana University Press.

Morris, E. (2009). Interview. In M. V. Beusekom, P. Ferrari, & J. Baichwal (Eds.), *Capturing reality: The art of documentary*. New York: First Run Features.

Mulvey, L. (1975). Visual pleasure and narrative cinema. *Screen, 16*, 6-18.

Nyhan, B., & Reifler, J. (2010). When corrections fail: The persistence of political misperceptions. *Political Behavior, 32*, 303-330.

Norris, A. E., & DeMarco, R. (2005). The experience of African American women living with HIV: Creating a prevention film for teens. *Journal of the Association of Nurses in AIDS Care, 16*(2), 32-39.

O'Rourke, R. (2001). Anya's movies. *Afterimage, 29*, 9.

Polanyi, M. (1966). *The tacit dimension*. Chicago, IL: University of Chicago.

Rabiger, M. (2009). *Directing the documentary* (5th ed.). Boston, MA: Focal Press.

Shirky, C. (2010). *Cognitive surplus: Creativity and generosity in a connected age*. New York: Penguin Press.

Stevens, B. (2009). Interview. In M. V. Beusekom, P. Ferrari, & J. Baichwal (Eds.), *Capturing reality: The art of documentary*. New York: First Run Features.

Twenge, J. M. (2013). Overwhelming evidence for generation me: A reply to Arnett. *Emerging Adulthood, 1*, 21-26.

Winston, B. (2002). *Media, technology and society: A history from the telegraph to the internet*. New York: Routledge.

Chapter 14: Approaches to evaluation: How to measure change when utilizing creative approaches

Jill M. Chonody

Introduction

An increasing need to show evidence of effective practice is a reality for many practitioners. Funders may require that practitioners show how their methods are creating change or improving the lives of those engaged at their agency or organization. Thus the funding needs and aims of the agency will likely guide the research questions and the methods used to answer those questions. For those practitioners who are not under this type of pressure, they may also want to know if their approaches are leading to change, as this is one aspect of ethical practice.

A variety of methods are available for collecting and analyzing data from the simple to complex. Depending on one's needs and training, outside researchers may be necessary to implement a full-scale investigation. Partnerships with researchers/academic faculty from a local university or institute may be one route for help with an evaluation. Grant writing and the inclusion of doctoral students/candidates or honor's students may be other avenues for involving university staff and faculty in a community-based project. A good place to start is with one question: "What do I want to know?" For example, the practitioner may want to know: "Have participants changed?" Naturally following this question may be: "If participants have changed, in what way have they changed?" Alternatively, the practitioner may want to know: "Does this program work?" or "Has the community responded to this project?" Once the primary research question has been formulated, the practitioner will then need to consider the best way to answer it.

The purpose of this chapter is to provide an overview of ways to evaluate interventions/activities and programs that utilize art or creative practices. This chapter is not meant to be comprehensive or give a step-by-step approach to evaluation. Rather, it is meant to provide a starting point for evaluative methods and give tips on where to go from here. Starting with further information on how *what* you want to know influences *how* you gather information to answer your research question leads to an overview of quantitative and qualitative methods of data collection, including design issues and data analysis. The way that the creative product fits into the research process is also an important consideration. A brief review of ways that art is incorporated into the research process is discussed, including art as illustration, art as a method of evaluation, and art as data. The benefits and potential challenges for each method are also presented.

Once the data are collected and analyzed, dissemination of the findings will also need to be considered. When creative outputs are part of the research process, the practitioner is in a better position for generating public engagement given that findings may be publicly displayed (e.g., performance, exhibition) to showcase innovative programs (Clark, 2012). Whether it is a report to a funding agency or a community event, the practitioner must closely weigh ethical issues surrounding participant consent for use of their creative product. This issue is discussed in the *Ethical Considerations* section near the end of this chapter as are practical tips for practitioners who want to initiate an evaluation. Concluding this chapter is a case example by Wernick and colleagues of how theater was used to address bullying, and the evaluation method that was used to assess their efforts.

Forming a Research Question

To create a good question, the practitioner must be very clear as to what objective s/he wishes to achieve. Care should be taken in conceiving what elements are investigated as this is reflected in the phrasing of the question and influences the methods. For example, if the practitioner wants to know if participants were happy with their participation in a creative endeavor, then the research question may be: "How happy were participants after participating in the intervention?" The use of how and the defining of the variable (re: happy) will limit the data that are needed to answer this question. If however, the practitioner wants to know how people felt as a result of their participation, then the question changes to something like, "How did you feel about your participation in the intervention?" These small shifts will shape the type of data collection methods that are utilized as well as what type of data that the practitioner will have at the end of the process. As stated previously, ask yourself: "What do I want to know?"

Quantitative Approaches

Quantitative methodology is vast, and as such, only a small scope can be presented herein. The primary focus of this section is geared toward data collection and includes considerations for measurement of outcomes. Given that approaches to quantitative analyses are dependent on sample size, number and type of variables included, and the type of statistical test, it is not possible to include a full discussion of analyses in this chapter. Moreover, training or assistance will likely be need if this is not already an area where the practitioner has experience. Nonetheless, a few simple ways to present the data are discussed below.

Design: Single-Systems

The basic elements of the research design are: When will the data be collected? From whom will it be collected? For most practice scenarios, information will be gathered from each participant. This information (e.g., data) is then typically used either to describe the individual or a group of individuals as a whole. This type of design is called single-systems design and is reviewed here. Most quantitative approaches to data collection require sampling methods and considerations of other issues, such as generalizability. For this approach, all those involved in the process would be asked to take part in the research process.

Single-systems designs are ideal if the practitioner is just looking to determine if there is change in the right direction (i.e., the individual is improving). In this approach, the practitioner gathers data by measuring (e.g., single-item indicator; discussed below) some personal attribute (e.g., self-confidence), before, during, and after intervention. The data are graphed for the individual(s) and visually inspected for positive change. For example, if a practitioner is working with a client to alleviate anxiety, then the practitioner could assess the level of anxiety throughout the process of intervention and track any changes.

This approach can also be applied when working with groups to determine if the group as a whole is exhibiting change and tracked in a similar fashion. After collecting information from each of the individual participants, these data could be averaged to give an indication of how the group is changing. Alternatively, the practitioner may collect data only twice for each participant—once prior to intervention and then again after the intervention. Individual graphs (discussed further below) for each participant could be compared to determine if change is going in the right direction. As in the example above, the practitioner would be seeking to know if anxiety decreased from the start of the intervention/program to the end of it. For further information on this type of approach to studying clients and client systems, see books on single-system design (one is provided in the *Recommended Readings and Resources* list at the end of the chapter).

Data Collection

Quantitative data are often collected by distributing surveys or questionnaires to a group of people, in this case, participants of a creative project or an individual client. A survey may contain standardized scales (see below for more discussion of these), such as a scale that measures self-esteem, along with basic demographic type questions (e.g., age, gender, etc.). Surveys are an easy way to collect a lot of data quickly and allows for comparison between participants because the same information is collected for each person. Moreover, this is an inexpensive way to collect information that also protects the confidentiality of the client.

Quantitative data can also be collected via observation. For example, a practitioner could count the number of crying spells that a participant has during an ongoing intervention to determine if a decrease occurs as a result of participation.

Measurement

Measurement of the targeted variable can be accomplished by a number of strategies. Again, the research question will shape the measurement strategy. The key to good measurement is twofold: 1) asking good questions, and 2) consistency in measurement over time. Quantitative data are limited by the questions that are asked; you can only know what you ask. Moreover, quantitative data cannot be compared if measurement strategies are changed between data collection points or across individuals/group; apples need to be compared to apples.

Standardized Instruments

Standardized instruments are scales that have been developed and tested by researchers to capture a complex concept or phenomenon (e.g., well-being, self-esteem, life satisfaction). These scales can be extremely useful because they offer a reliable and valid approach to gathering information. For example, if the practitioner would like to determine if self-esteem improved as the result of participation in a creative program, what aspects of behavior, attitudes, or values will be measured to capture the notion of "self-esteem"? A standardized scale of self-esteem resolves this issue given that it has a number of items that have been developed to represent "self-esteem." However, standardized scales do not exist for everything that practitioners may want to know or they may not be readily accessible. Fischer and Corcoran (2007) offer several volumes that contain scales for individuals (including both children and adults), couples, and families (see *Recommended Readings and Resources* at the end of the chapter for the full reference).

Single-Item Indicators

In addition to or instead of a standardized scale, the practitioner may want to create a single-item indicator to measure change. For example, the practitioner could ask participants to indicate on a scale of 1 to 10 their degree of depression. This item then could be repeated to the clients at key intervals during the intervention to measure changes and determine if the change is occurring in the direction that the practitioner anticipated. These data points can be graphed, averaged across participants, or presented as frequencies—or some combination of these. Furthermore, when working individually with a client, the practitioner can utilize the client's language in the creation of the indicator. For example, if a client describes his mood as "down in the dumps," then the single-item indicator might be: "On a scale of 1 to 7, how down in the dumps have you felt over the past week?"

The response range for single-item indicators should be no more than seven options if each option is named (e.g., 1=strongly disagree, 2=moderately disagree and so on). If the scale is simply anchored (i.e., bipolar adjectives at each end, such as 1=not depressed and 10=very depressed), then a ten-point scale is likely the upper limit. Most standardized scales have recommended response ranges.

Observation

Direct observation is another way to measure change. For example, the practitioner may want to know if the number of angry outbursts that a child exhibits during group sessions have decreased. Once "angry outburst" is fully defined (e.g., does this include yelling? Screaming? Fighting?), then the practitioner needs to create a way to count the occurrence(s) during a particular time frame, such as a group session. Accurate counts rely on clearly defined variables. For example, if the child gets angry, does that count as an "outburst?" What if she starts yelling immediately after the group session? This can be a good way to capture behavioral changes, but parameters for measurement must be defined prior to counting to create accuracy in the data.

Data Analysis

As mentioned above, visual analysis of graphs can be used to track changes. This is a simple and straightforward way for practitioners to monitor individual and/or group change. Along the x-axis, time is tracked and along the y-axis, the variable of interest is measured (e.g., emotional expression). Figure 1 provides an example of how one of these graphs may look. The graphs are monitored to determine if change is occurring in the direction that the practitioner intended. For example, if a client were completing a scale at each weekly session regarding her anxiety for the week (higher scores indicating greater anxiety), then the practitioner would want to see that the line on the graph is declining. This strategy can be used with any of the above approaches to measurement (e.g., standardized scales), and these graphs may be used in charts or become part of reports.

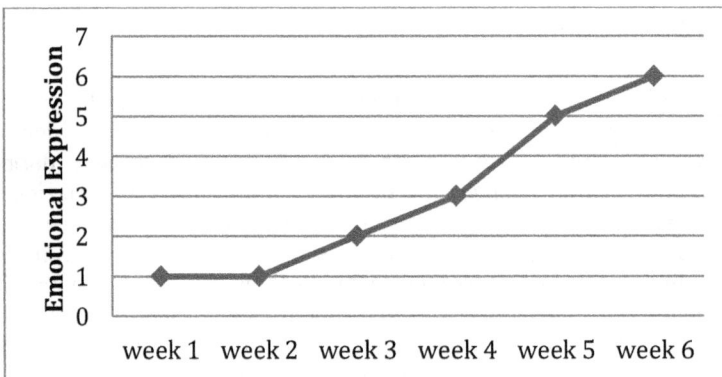

Figure 1

Another simple way to present quantitative data to funders or within reports is simply to show the frequencies and averages within the data. For example, the practitioner can indicate the number of participants who showed improvement in mood after participating in the program. Signs of improvement can also be illustrated through group frequencies. For example, the practitioner may report: "30% of the group indicated improved mood after participating in the project."

The practitioner can also present the mean (i.e., the average) change that occurred for a participant or participants. For example, if on average a participant scored low on a measure self-worth before the intervention, and it was higher after the intervention, then this information could be easily included alongside frequencies or other counts. Alternatively, a practitioner may want to collect information regarding participant satisfaction. For example, if a mural was created in the community and the practitioner sought to determine if community members were satisfied with it, then the practitioner could ask members: "On a scale of 1 to 5 (5 being completely satisfied), how satisfied are you with the mural?" The practitioner could present the findings as a frequency (e.g., 75% of the people who answered the survey were satisfied with the mural) or as a mean (e.g., on average, community satisfaction with the mural was a 4.2 out of 5). More complex approaches to data analyses (e.g., regression, analysis of variance) are not included here, but a multitude of other analyses are possible depending on the type of data collected, the sample size, the number of variables, and the research questions. Outside consultancy may be necessary if the practitioner is not trained in these more complex analyses.

Benefits and Potential Challenges

The primary benefit of quantitative approaches is that they can allow for comparison over time given that the same measures are used consistently with new groups. Objective measures not only standardize assessment, but also provide some protection against practitioner interpretation. Similarly, they can also allow for comparison across groups and individuals through the use of statistical analyses. Furthermore, it is easy to collect data from a large group of people in a short time frame with quantitative methods.

The key challenge in quantitative approaches is that the analyses may require statistical expertise, which the practitioner may not be trained to do. Thus, outside help may be needed to fully implement a large scale, quantitative research study. Similarly, large samples sizes are required for certain kinds of analyses, which may not be available or difficult to access.

Qualitative Approaches

Qualitative approaches, like quantitative methods, are useful with individuals, groups, community, and program evaluation, but the method and the analyses of any research project depends on your research question. While there are many approaches to qualitative data collection and analyses, a few are offered here to give a sense of where to start.

What is the "data" in qualitative research?

The data in qualitative research are the words or text that is gathered from participants. These words may be spoken such as in an interview, come from case notes, or be gathered by observation of the environment (i.e., field notes). Any document can be a source of qualitative data, but for many practitioners, they will likely seek to gather information—or data—directly from participants through interviews and focus groups (discussed below), which are audio-recorded and then transcribed for data analyses.

Design

Two basic types of designs that may be employed in qualitative data collection are the case study and a group design. A case study presents the narrative of one particular participant of an intervention or one community, neighborhood, organization, or program. The type of case study along with the kind of intervention that has been implemented, the target of that effort, and the research question will determine the type of data that will need to be gathered. If the focus is on one client for example, then the case study will seek to illustrate those aspects of the story that showcase where the client began, how the process of creative intervention affected her/him, and the results of the process for that individual. Case studies represent a way to create a deep understanding of a particular client and can be a particularly powerful way to present the program to others. Case studies could be collected over time on a number of program participants and then later subjected to content analysis (see below) to elucidate the themes that emerge from the program over time.

Alternatively, a group design would seek to learn about an issue by hearing the perspective of multiple people who have knowledge/experience about that topic. For example, a practitioner who works with homeless youth in a shelter setting may want to learn more about the lived experience of her/his clients by implementing a photovoice project (see Chapter 2 for more information on photovoice). Through a series of photo-shoots, interviews and group discussions about the photographs, the experience of homelessness, and their perspective on the project, the practitioner gains insight by seeking out the communalities and exceptions during the data analysis process.

Data Collection

While case notes and other documents (e.g., stories that participants write) may used as data, the main focus in this section is how to collect additional information from participants regarding their experience/perspective on the program/intervention or a particular social issue (e.g., mental health stigma).

Interviews

Interviews are used to gather information from participants on a one-to-one basis and offer varying degrees of depth (e.g., ethnographic interviewing). Typically, participants are interviewed about a few topics/issues in depth, but their entire background is not the focus. For example, participants of a program may be individually interviewed to explore their reaction to using a creative method as an outlet for emotional expression along with the degree to which they felt satisfied by the process. However, interviewing may also be used to create in-depth case studies as well. For example, if a case study about a community is generated, then interviews with key people from that community are essential.

Focus Groups

Focus groups also provide a level of depth to the information gathered and are used to explore a topic through group discussion (e.g., an exploration of a particular experience). The level of depth may actually be enhanced by the exchanges between and among participants, but requires participants to be willing to discuss information in front of one another. A downside is that some voices become less explored than would have been the case with individual interviews.

This type of data collection is useful in evaluation and other types of research. For example, a series of focus groups might be used to discuss participants' experience with the program, the creative approach, and any changes that have occurred as a result of participation. This approach provides the researcher an efficient way to gather a range of information in short time. Group facilitation skills are key as is asking good questions. The practitioner should think about what questions to ask and how these questions will help to answer the overall research question prior to initiating a focus group.

Data Analysis

Although there are many approaches to data analysis within the qualitative methods, only two are presented here as they offer useful ways for thinking about how words can be analyzed.

Thematic and Content Analysis

Thematic analysis typically focuses on determining the major findings from a set of data or the primary themes that emerge whereas content analysis seeks to code and then count the occurrences of specific categories within the data (Corbin & Strauss, 2008). These approaches can be used in concert with one another or alone.

To create the themes or codes, the practitioner immerses her/himself in the data. In other words, all the content that has been collected is thoroughly reviewed before attempting the formal analysis. As codes are created, the practitioner engages in a constant comparison between occurrences in the data to look for similarities and differences. The final themes or codes that are found in the data are then presented along with illustrative quotes. For example, if one of the themes found was that participants felt proud of their dance performance, then this theme would be presented along with a quote, such as, "I felt very pleased by our performance, and I felt so proud when the audience clapped and cheered."

Summarizing and creating themes based on the information that has been gathered can be fairly straightforward process (see Braun & Clark, 2007 for further information of this approach; the full reference is available at the end of the chapter) and offer a wealth of information about the program/intervention. These methods can also be used in conjunction with quantitative methods (i.e., mixed methods approach) to gather different kinds of information. For example, a mixed methods design may entail a questionnaire with a combination of closed and open-ended questions or a short survey along with a focus group. Research questions will guide the methods in addition to resources and needs of the agency/program.

Benefits and Potential Challenges

The chief benefit of qualitative data collection is the rich level of detail that comes directly from the participants' perspective. When data are collected within the context of an interview or focus group, follow-up questions can be posed and shifts in the information that is collected can occur based on data already collected. Moreover, this type of data collection occurs in a setting that is already familiar to both participants and practitioners, that is, having a conversation in groups or one-on-one. Similarly, it offers some flexibility for participants in that they are not constrained by standardized scales and thus they can more fully explain their thoughts and feelings.

The primary drawback to qualitative research is that it can be time consuming. Since interviews and focus groups are typically recorded so that the audio can be reviewed later and used for data analysis, transcription is labor intensive, but necessary for a full immersion in the data. Relatedly, identifying overarching themes may be challenging in some datasets, and explaining the findings is not always straightforward. Lastly, if the interviews/focus groups are conducted by the practitioner who also implemented the program, then social pressure on the participants may force them to be overly positive, complementary, or confirmatory in their responses.

Art and Evaluation

> Visual representations of experience—in photographs, performance art, and other media—can enable others to see as a participant sees (Riessman, 2008, p. 142).

Art products can be used in a number of ways in evaluation. Art can be used to illustrate the creativity of a project/program or as a way to showcase what the participants learned through the process or how they changed. Art can also be used as the primary method for investigating the value of a program or as the primary source of data, which requires some level of art interpretation to uncover its layered meaning. Each of these approaches is briefly reviewed below.

Art as Illustration

Art as illustration of a program or change process is not a research method or an approach to analysis, but rather, is a way to represent research findings from studies that include creative practices. Thus, other data are collected to determine the outcome, and the art product is the showcase of those findings. In some instances, the art products are also shown in a public forum (e.g., performances, gallery exhibit), and this may offer an additional layer of intervention. For example, in Chapter 2, a description of how photography was incorporated into a research project that explored adolescents' perceptions of community is provided. The images that were created by the youth became illustrative of the themes that were generated from the qualitative analyses of the focus groups that were held throughout the project. Participants also chose several of their photographs for an open house display of their creative work where friends and family were in attendance. The use of images in this way adds to the data in a number of ways, namely "images put a face on statistical data" (Harper, 2008, p. 187).

Beyond this, the images provide a context for the data, illustrate interrelated ideas or concepts, help viewers connect with the findings, and may even challenge previously held assumptions (Harper, 2008). Nonetheless, the images are secondary to the research process and while they are "important to the text…the visual dimension is integrated into the research" (Harper, 2008, p. 187). Dissemination of research findings—to funders, in public forums, or in professional publishing capacities—may have a greater impact when creative aspects of the program are used to illustrate the findings; however, ethical issues should be carefully considered. Some of these issues are explored later in the chapter.

Art as a Method for Evaluation

The use of art as a method for collecting data can help the practitioner to better understand the crux of participants' experience, "because it helps to access the feelings and emotions embedded in the experience and—through imagery, poetic form, or dramatic reenactment—capture the power and meaning of that experience" (Simons & McCormack, 2007, p. 301). Thus, the art/creative product (e.g., photograph, song, etc.) is the data that are used for evaluation. While this is perhaps a more abstract way to think about research, it does not need to run counter to other approaches, and a group method or individual approach can be employed. For example, the practitioner could have participants create a mural or use found/re-purposed objects to represent their experience in the program. Alternatively, individual participants could be asked to reveal what they will take away from the program through the use of a creative medium, such as dance or poetry (Simons & McCormack, 2007). In other words, an artistic expression can be used to evaluate another creative product, but the exact way that the participant chooses to express her/his feelings is left completely up to the individual.

Further inclusion of creative arts in the research process can help advance the methods for how art is used in practice. Moreover, the use of art and creative activities can highlight "the essential values of a program" (Simons & McCormack, 2007, p. 294). The use of art as evaluation offers a different way of knowing, which frees the practitioner from the traditional holds of the research process, such as coding, categorizing, and statistical analyses (Simons & McCormack, 2007). Designing and evaluating practice through art will stretch the practitioner to develop creative studies to explore how these creative works symbolize experience and growth.

Art as Data: Interpretation of Art Products

There are multiple ways to use creative works as data, including identifying trends on blogs (Runte, 2008), using qualitative data to stage a theatrical performance (Donmoyer & Donmoyer, 2008), or interpreting photographs as data (Collier & Collier, 1986). Likewise, art interpretation can be used as a way to generate data. Interpretation of art as the mode of inquiry can include both how the product was created (i.e., the process of creating art) and an interpretation of the art product (i.e., visual analysis) by different audiences (Riessman, 2008).

In terms of process, practitioners may seek to understand how participants went about creating their art products. Whether it is film or poetry, the meaning associated with the process and product may be ascertained by discussing them with the creators. The practitioner may inquire as to how the composition came to be as it is. Through this exploration, insights regarding *why* this came to be will be revealed. This method of exploration is particularly applicable to mediums such as photography (Riessman, 2008); however, it is readily transferrable to storytelling, film, painting, drawing, sculpture, mural/street art, and repurposed objects. This approach could also be applied to performance-based arts when participants are choreographing the dance, creating the music, or writing the play. Participants can be interviewed regarding their choices and the meaning behind those decisions. Thus, the art itself is the data. Some questions that may be helpful for this process of exploration:

1. What did you intend for this mean when you began making it? Has that changed? If so, how?
2. How should this creative product be read? What other interpretations might be made?
3. Is this product connected to other work? Or perhaps text?
4. How did you decide upon this composition? Does it represent other aspects of you, your work, or your journey? (adapted from Riessman, 2008, p. 143-144).

An alternative approach to using art as data relies on interpretation of the product. For example, one might begin with just noting initial impressions and "intellectual speculations," which may lead to specific categories that can be used for counting or measuring (Collier & Collier, 1986, p. 172). The practitioner might begin with a two-part question: 1) "What do I see?" and 2) "How do I know?" (Collier & Collier, 1986, p. 172). For example, the practitioner may consider issues of composition, subject, and light or review a series of images created over a period of time while noting these impressions, feelings, and perceptions of the artwork. Content analysis techniques can be utilized once the notes and interpretations are complete.

On the other hand, visual elements could be counted to determine the frequency of their occurrence (Rose, 2007). For example, if working with a group of adolescents with depression, the practitioner may come to realize that a participant focuses on very dark images in his work. Thus, when analyzing the images over time, the practitioner would count the frequency that this occurs at specific time points to establish if this changes over time. This approach may also be applied if analyzing a large group of images for many participants. The practitioner will need to develop a set of codes or categories based on the images, and then each one will need to be placed within in it. The practitioner can then look for change over time or simply count how many images fall within each of the categories (Rose, 2007).

Each of these suggestions offers the practitioner significant food for thought when considering the use of art as data. A final aspect to consider when incorporating creative practices into the research process is that an outcome-based approach to determine if project/program "works" will likely include the evaluation or interpretation of art products. Art interpretation may seek to determine if change in content or meaning has occurred. Visual products (e.g., street art, film, photography, sculpture, painting, drawing, found objects) are evaluated either throughout the program or period of intervention or at the beginning and again at the end. Similarly, document analysis or narrative analysis can offer a similar process when words are the creative outlet. Storytelling, journaling, and other writings (including poetry and fiction) can be assessed for individual growth and change during the period of intervention. On the other hand, art interpretation can be joined with quantitative or qualitative methods to generate a multifaceted evaluation. For example, the addition of measuring change in another way, such as a simple question posed periodically throughout the intervention/program (e.g., on a scale of 1 to 10 with 10 being the best, how would you rate your mood?) may complement the art interpretation process. Moreover, interviews could be used to explore the practitioner's interpretations with the art creator. This process may reveal further insights about process and product.

In sum, art products and creativity can be incorporated in a variety of ways in the research process. Art as illustration and participant driven interpretation are likely the most direct ways to include creative products in the process of evaluation. Practitioner interpretation simply represents an alternative approach and is not something that should be thought of as inherent to the process. Moreover, it can create other issues, both in terms of data and participant empowerment. These issues are explored in *Ethical Considerations*.

Benefits and Potential Challenges

The main benefit of art as illustration is that it showcases the creativity of individual participants and the overall program/project. It can also communicate significant themes in a way that can resonate more than words. An important drawback is that images can create confusion for the viewer or may be used superficially to promote the agency/program. Careful use, including permission from the artist, is a vital aspect of using art as illustration.

Using art as the method of evaluation has the central benefit that it represents a different way of knowing, which can generate a novel way to understand the process of change (Simmons & McCormack, 2007). One issue related to using art as the evaluation is directly related to its advantage—standardization. If ongoing assessment of a program is part of a long-term plan, then the lack of comparable data across many groups can be problematic. For example, the practitioner may have a different theme for every evaluation, which in turn, would mean that if 100 participants had completed the program, then 100 different themes would need to be represented. This can be a challenge when reporting outcomes to funders, agency managers, and government officials. The essential difficulty of using art as evaluation is its translation into words (McNiff, 2007). Knowing how to translate art into language, and represent the art appropriately, can be a challenge for both the practitioner-researcher and the participant-artist. Allowing time, review, and revision may help the practitioner achieve the goal of representing the process and product through narrative descriptions. A final issue to consider is the possible reaction of participants. Many people feel uncomfortable expressing themselves artistically for fear that their work will be judged harshly (Simons & McCormack, 2007). Reassurance that the purpose of the activity is about process, not product, may help individuals to overcome their fear.

The primary benefit of art interpretation is that the change is visually represented and illustrated. For example, if working with individuals who have experienced trauma, a change in the use of color may be noteworthy. A move from only using black and gray to represent the self to the introduction of color may show movement away from those troubling experiences. On the other hand, one of the key challenges for art interpretation is that one needs to be skilled at this process because misinterpretation could be a likely outcome. Relatedly, practitioner-based interpretation can rob the participant of her/his voice—the very thing that art gives back to people. Using interviewing and member checking (i.e., reviewing results with participants to clarify and check findings) to determine if interpretation is consistent with the participant's perspective may be a way to diminish this possibility.

Alternatively, art interpretation may be challenging for participants. It can be difficult to express in words the meaning and significance of creative products. The use of specific questions to guide the conversation may facilitate the process. If the practitioner is doing the interpretation, then it is possible that the art has not been truly represented at all. McNiff (2004) asks, "When will we realize that interpretations of art are the projections of those who make them?" Perhaps a balanced approach of practitioner interpretation alongside participant interpretation would produce a better process and a more accurate product. Moreover, the power imbalance between participant and practitioner can unduly influence the interpretation. In other words, the participant may think that the practitioner is the expert, and therefore, knows what the art product means instead of oneself as creator of that product (McNiff, 2004).

Ethical Considerations

Informed consent is an important ethical consideration when conducting research. First, participants need to feel that they can chose to participate (or not) as well as change their mind at will in regard to their continued involvement in a research study. Second, participants need to be fully informed about what they are going to be asked to do and if it involves any risk. Third, consent is also related to dissemination of their creative products. If these works are intended for use in reports, websites, published manuscripts, newspaper/magazine articles, or exhibited in public forums or spaces, then participant consent should be garnered for each use. Displaying or reproducing participant artwork may have a number of implications, including "relinquish[ing] control of how those images are made and interpreted, and, especially in the case of online display, potentially re-used by unknown viewers" (Clark, 2012, p. 23).

One way to address this issue is to create a detailed consent form for art products. In a photovoice project, Chonody, Ferman, Martin, and Amitrai-Welsh (2013) carefully considered this issue with their adolescent participants. First, each participant was given a printed contact sheet with all of her/his digital images as thumbnails and asked to cross through any image that they would not want to be used under any context. Since the project involved youth under the age of 18, none of the images of other participants or self-images were used either. Next, the consent form was distributed, which included a detailed list of the places that images may be used (e.g., a website, academic journal, professional conference, and newspaper). Participants indicated which of these forums, if any, that their images could be displayed. Then parental consent was sought. It was important to the research team that participants retained control over their work and its use.

Practitioners must be mindful of the ways in which their research is presented. There can be a tendency toward only including the "juicy stuff," and this may misrepresent not only the findings, but also the participants themselves (Siding et al., 2008, p. 465). Misrepresentation can lead to (un)intentional promotion of stereotypes, stigma, or invoke pity or even degradation. Participants may have real concerns about misrepresentation or more likely, unfavorable representation (Siding et al., 2008).

> When research results are presented as art, and public access to the work is both enabled and deliberately arranged, our recontextualizations of research participants' stories and lives become audible, visible, felt by them, in visceral and potentially lasting ways. To the extent that we have objectified them, they will know this objectification and experience it in public (Siding et al., 2008, p. 465).

Furthermore, practitioners need to carefully consider how best to protect participants' confidentiality. Using anonymous surveys (with a number to track individuals, if needed) are one way to protect the client's private information if the practitioner is collecting quantitative data. In qualitative research, confidentiality is something that needs to be discussed in focus groups, but it cannot be guaranteed. For example, if one participant reveals some private information during the focus group, then there is no way to ensure that the information does not leave that room given that other participants are involved in the process. During transcription of the qualitative data (interviews or focus groups), participants' names can be changed to pseudonyms to protect participants' confidentiality. This is also important when reporting information to funders, within reports, or in presentations. When working with certain mediums, the protection of identity can become problematic, especially photographs and film (Clark, 2012), but also drawing, painting, and sculpting, if a participant has a particular style. While techniques may be employed to protect the identity of an individual, such as pixelating faces, this may run contrary to the aims of the project; that is the creation of art (Clark, 2012).

Tips for Practitioners

1. **Consider contacting a local university for possible collaborations.** Academic or research faculty may be willing to help with program evaluation or community assessment. Search departmental websites such as social work, nursing, health, psychology, public policy, political

science, or related disciplines. Faculty often have their research interests listed next to their name along with their contact details. Some faculty members may do pro bono work, write a grant to do the work depending on available funding sources, or even just give some advice about the project.

2. **Before beginning a research project that includes data collection, check with the agency/organization leaders.** A formal review of the research plan may be necessary. For example, universities require that all research proposals (even community based research) be evaluated by their internal Institutional Review Board or an equivalent ethics board. Primary schools also typically require a similar process. If working with children under the age of 18, *parental consent* and *participant assent* are typically necessary for conducting research. Again, consider collaborations with academics/researchers to help sort through the complexities of conducting a study with children (or other vulnerable populations, such as people with cognitive impairment).

3. **Consider a simple approach to evaluation.** One measure of change (e.g., well-being) can be given before the intervention (or program) and then again after the intervention. Then simply compare the two scores to determine if the change is in the right direction. This approach is common when working with individuals (e.g., single- systems design) and can be adapted for groups—either to see if the group changed as whole or if the individuals within the group changed (or both). Alternatively, a focus group can be conducted with participants after the intervention to elicit feedback on how the intervention impacted them, and the themes from the data can be summarized.

4. **Consider using survey monkey.** If data are being collected from a large group of people located in various communities, internet-based sureys are a convenient way to collect this information. Free accounts are available if the survey is short, and the software is easy to use (view at: https://www.surveymonkey.com/home/). Sometimes Internet based surveys can reduce the number of people who will complete it, but it may be a better alternative to direct mailings.

5. **Collect information from participants as they start the program or the intervention.** This may be simple information, such as "What do you hope to achieve by participating in this project?" Or "How would you rate your mood on a scale of 1 to 10?" Funding issues and evidence informed practice are increasingly more pressing and showing that a program has merit in terms of change may be necessary.

6. **When working with the community, consider using multiple methods to collect data.** Perhaps hold some initial forums with focus groups to gather more information about a problem or issue that concerns community members and to garner their perspective on it, including ways to address it and feedback on what may be proposed by the practitioner. Surveys may be used to collect information from a broader sample of the community and can be based on the information gathered through focus groups. Once a project or program is

implemented, use evaluation forms or follow-up focus groups to determine what effects it has had on the community.

7. **When working with groups, consider using an evaluation feedback form.** Collecting information on how the program can be expanded or improved is important. It can be used in conjunction with research about how the program created change and will facilitate ways to tweak the approach that will strengthen its impact.

8. **When using art interpretation, carefully balance the role of the practitioner, the participant, and the focus of the project/evaluation.** If the practitioner decides to interpret art products as part of the research process, discuss those interpretations with participants. Alternatively, consider having someone else conduct an initial interview or focus group with participants to gather their interpretations. Then the practitioner can compare her/his findings with the data collected from participants. As a final step, the practitioner could go back to participants for a discussion of both sets of results.

9. **Create a detailed consent form for reproduction or use of creative products generated in the project for research purposes.** Participants' right to control their artwork is essential to personal empowerment and ethical practice. This includes any items that may be made from their artwork to produce money for the program. For example, creating a calendar of the drawings of children participating in a social skills group for the expressed purposes of re-funding the program should still obtain the consent of the parents and the assent of the child.

10. **Use your creativity when compiling reports!** When using art as a method of evaluation, reports and presentations to funders or agency leaders will likely need to include written words and narratives. In writing those reports, the practitioner should consider ways to "enrich the text with images, cartoons, graphics, dialogue, brief narratives, voice, vignettes, cameos, and color" to present the findings (Simons & McCormack, 2007, p. 306).

Recommended Readings and Resources

Braun, V., & Clarke, V. (2007). Using thematic analysis in psychology. *Qualitative Research in Psychology, 3,* 77-101.

DiNoia, J., & Tripodi, T. (2008). *Single-case design for clinical social workers* (2nd ed.). Baltimore, MD: NASW Press.

Fischer, J., & Corcoran, K. (2007). *Measures for clinical practice and research: A sourcebook, Volume 1: Couples, Families, and Children* (4th ed.). New York: Oxford University Press.

Fischer, J., & Corcoran, K. (2007). *Measures for clinical practice and research: A sourcebook, Volume 2: Adults* (4th ed.). New York: Oxford University Press.

Kapp, S. A., & Anderson, G. R. (2010). *Agency-based program evaluation: Lessons from practice.* Thousand Oaks, CA: Sage.

Knowles, J. G., & Cole, A. L. (Eds.). (2008). *Handbook of arts in qualitative research: Perspectives, methodologies, examples, and issues*. Thousand Oaks, CA: Sage.

Leavy, P. (2009). *Method meets art: Arts-based research practice*. New York: Guilford.

Prosser, J. (Ed.). (1998). *Image-based research: A sourcebook for qualitative researchers*. London: Routledge-Falmer.

Rose, G. (2007). *Visual methodologies: An introduction to the interpretation of visual materials* (2nd ed.). London: Sage.

Royse, D. (2011). *Research methods in social work* (6th ed.). Belmont, CA: Cengage.

References

Chase, S. (2008). Narrative inquiry: Multiple lenses, approaches, voices. In N. K. Denzin & Y. S. Lincoln (Eds.), *Collecting and interpreting qualitative materials* (3rd ed., pp. 57-94). Los Angeles, CA: Sage.

Chonody, J. M., Ferman, B., Amitrani-Welsh, J., & Martin, T. (2013). Violence through the eyes of youth: A photovoice exploration. *Journal of Community Psychology, 41,* 84-101.

Corbin, J., & Strauss, A. (2008). Strategies for qualitative data analysis. In *Basics of qualitative research: Techniques and procedures for developing grounded theory* (3rd ed., pp. 65-86). Los Angeles, CA: Sage.

Clark, A. (2012). Visual ethics in a contemporary landscape. In S. Pink (Ed.), *Advances in visual methodology* (pp. 17-36). London: Sage.

Collier, J., Jr., & Collier, M. (1986). Principles of visual research. In *Visual anthropology: Photography as a research method* (pp. 161-174). Albuquerque, NM: University of New Mexico Press.

Donmoyer, R., & Donmoyer, J. Y. (2008). Readers' theater as data display strategy. In J. G. Knowles & A. L Cole. (Eds.), *Handbook of the arts in qualitative research: Perspectives, methodologies, examples, and issues* (pp. 209-224). Thousand Oaks, CA: Sage.

Harper, D. (2008). What's new visually. In N. K. Denzin & Y. S. Lincoln (Eds.), *Collecting and interpreting qualitative materials* (3rd ed., pp. 185-204). Los Angeles, CA: Sage.

McNiff, S. (2007). Art-based research. In J. Gary & A. L. Cole (Eds.), *Handbook of arts in qualitative research: Perspectives, methodologies, examples, and issues* (pp. 29-40). Thousand Oaks, CA: Sage.

McNiff, S. (2004). The interpretation of imagery. In *Art heals: How creativity cures the soul* (pp. 75-81). Boston, MA: Shambhala.

Riessman, C. K. (2008). Visual Analysis. In *Narrative methods for the human sciences* (pp. 141-182). Thousand Oaks, CA: Sage.

Rose, G. (2007). Content analysis: Counting what you (think you) see. In *Visual methodologies: An introduction to the interpretation of visual materials* (2nd ed., pp. 54-68). London: Sage.

Runte, R. (2008). Blogs. In J. Gary & A. L. Cole (Eds.), *Handbook of arts in qualitative research: Perspectives, methodologies, examples, and issues* (pp. 313-322). Thousand Oaks, CA: Sage.

Simmons, H., & McCormack, B. (2007). Integrating arts-based inquiry in evaluation methodology: Opportunities and challenges. *Qualitative Inquiry, 13*, 292-311.

Sinding, C., Gray, R., & Nisker, J. (2008). In J. Gary & A. L. Cole (Eds.), *Handbook of arts in qualitative research: Perspectives, methodologies, examples, and issues* (pp. 459-460). Thousand Oaks, CA: Sage.

Case Application: Evaluating an LGBTQQ-Youth Led Intervention that uses Theater and Dialogue

Laura J. Wernick, Adrienne B. Dessel, Alex Kulick, & Louis F. Graham

Riot Youth and Gayrilla Theater

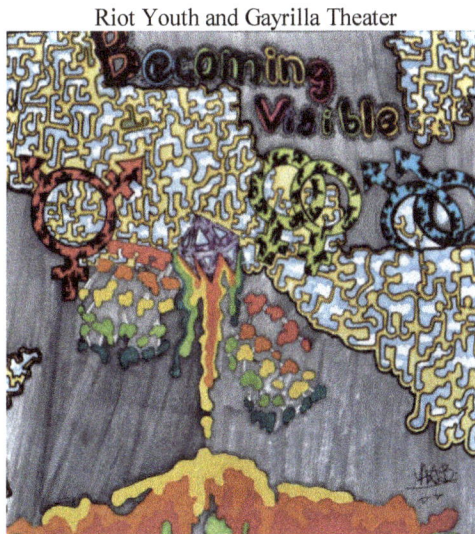

Title: *Becoming Visible: Climate Survey Toolkit.*
Photo by: Neutral Zone.

Riot Youth is a youth-driven lesbian, gay, bisexual, transgender, queer, questioning, and allied (LGBTQQA) program based out of the *Neutral Zone* in Ann Arbor, Michigan. The program provides a safe space for youth leaders to build community and organize for social justice. In 2007, using a participatory action research framework, *Riot Youth* created a school climate survey and disseminated it to nearly 1,200 students in four high schools in Ann Arbor.

Through theater games, discussions of the climate survey findings, and personal storytelling, *Riot Youth* worked with a scriptwriter to develop a performance called "Gayrilla," which comprised a series of skits designed to build knowledge, raise awareness, and begin conversations among middle and high school students. Following the performances, students were separated into smaller groups for youth-facilitated dialogues. These dialogues were an opportunity to share experiences, ask questions, voice concerns, and develop skills to take action. The dialogues interweaved discussions about identities, including sexual orientation, gender identity, race, disability, and appearance.

Designing and Distributing the Evaluation Instrument

Youth were interested in understanding how participation in *Gayrilla* impacted students, and they decided to systematically survey participants using a pre-/post-test. Youth leaders and a team of university researchers collaboratively developed survey items, which included demographic questions, quantitative items, and "write-in" responses. Demographics included grade, race, gender, and sexual orientation. The pre-test included items assessing frequency of witnessing anti-LGBTQQ harassment and self-reported existing intervention behaviors when witnessing anti-LGBTQQ bullying/harassment. Respondents were also asked two open-ended questions about why they had or had not intervened.

Three paired items were used on the pre- and post-tests to measure changes related to participation in the intervention: desire to intervene when witnessing anti-LGBTQQ harassment, confidence to successfully do so, and willingness to advocate for social justice for LGBTQQ people. Paired open-ended items inquired about awareness of homophobia/transphobia and how they decided whether or not to intervene. Youth leaders wrote some items and others were adapted from standardized scales.

Youth distributed pre-test surveys before the performance, and post-test surveys were collected in a sealed envelope following the dialogue. Surveys were assigned a numerical code to anonymously match pre- and post-test surveys.

Analyses and Using Findings

Analyses of the surveys showed a statistically significant difference from the pre- to post-tests on all three measures: desire to intervene, confidence to intervene, and likelihood to advocate. An exploration of the write-in responses yielded deeper insight into how and why students were changed through participation in *Gayrilla*. Finally, our analyses also suggested that the intervention was significantly more effective in increasing White students' desire to intervene against bullying when compared to students of Color, and slightly more effective with regards to confidence to intervene.

Youth leaders took these findings to school administrators to demonstrate the effectiveness of their intervention and to advocate for *Gayrilla* performances and post-performance dialogues to be conducted in more schools. One school administrator, who had been previously resistant to having students participate, explicitly cited the evaluation findings as a reason to change their decision. Moreover, the youth used these findings to plan revisions to the script and additional strategies for future interventions, and the organization utilized these findings for reports to funders and new grant applications, which would help to secure funding that enables the continuation of a youth-driven arts-based intervention strategy. Finally, the university team has produced two academic papers and given national presentations to share these findings with a broader audience.

Resources and Recommended Readings

Riot Youth. (2013). *Becoming visible: A project of Riot Youth at the Neutral Zone.* Ann Arbor, MI: Neutral Zone. Available at: http://www.neutral-zone.org/programs/1070/gayrilla-becoming-visible.

Riot Youth. (2009). *The Riot Youth Climate Survey of Ann Arbor public high schools: Report of findings.* Ann Arbor, MI: Neutral Zone. Available at: http://www.neutral-zone.org/programs/679/riot-youth-presents-its-school-climate-survey.

Wernick, L. J., Dessel, A. B., Kulick, A., & Graham, L. F. (2013). LGBTQQ youth creating change: Developing allies against bullying through performance and dialogue. *Children & Youth Services Review, 35,* 1576-1586.

Wernick, L. J., Kulick, A., & Inglehart, M. H. (2013). Factors predicting student intervention when witnessing anti-LGBTQ harassment: The influence of peers, teachers and climate. *Children & Youth Services Review, 35,* 296-301.

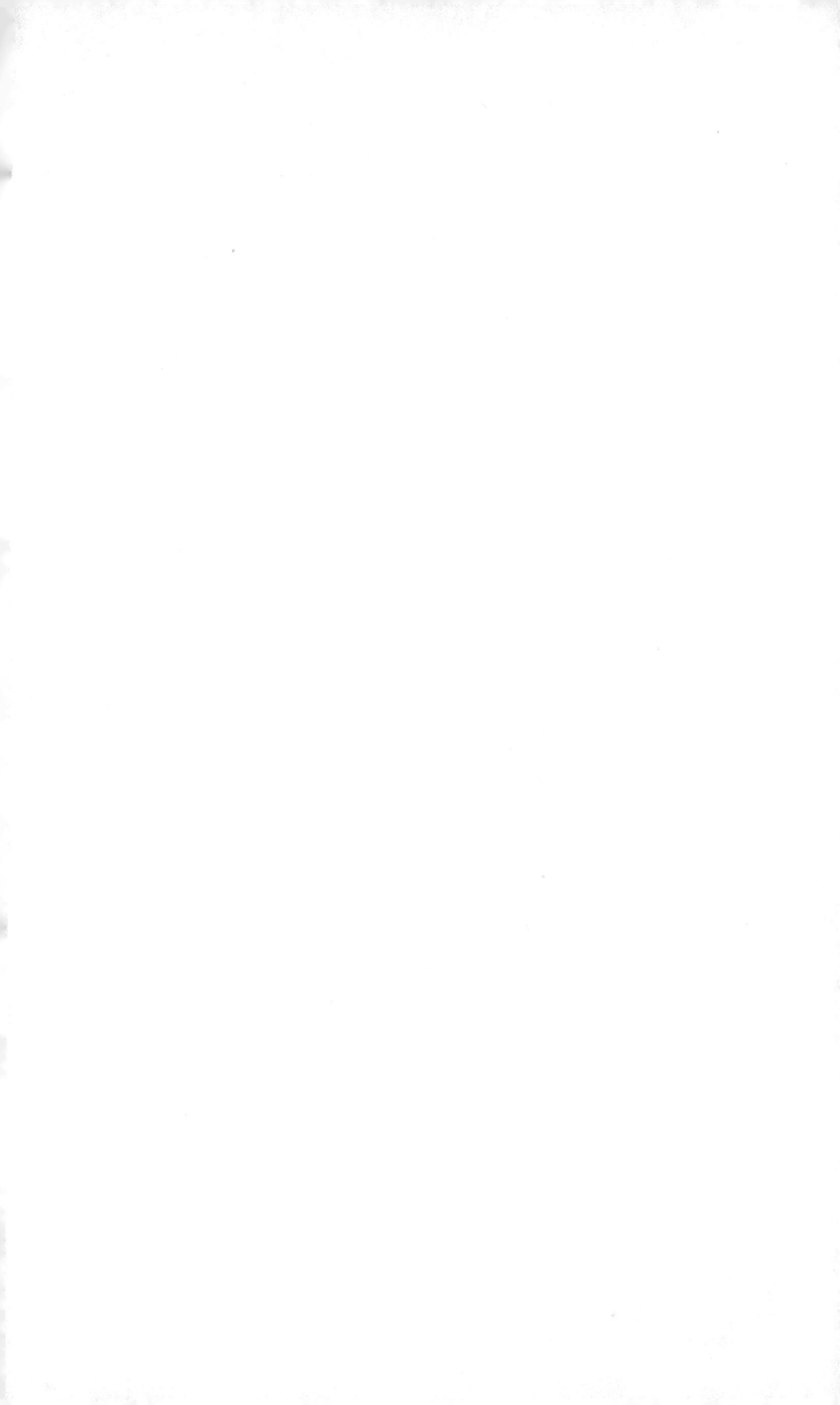

www.ingramcontent.com/pod-product-compliance
Lightning Source LLC
Chambersburg PA
CBHW072105040426
42334CB00042B/2345